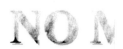

NO MATTER WHAT

Finding the answers to dealing with a life changing diagnosis to help Steven who suffers from Autism

Sandy Howarth

Sandy Howarth

Published by
Chipmunkapublishing
PO Box 6872
Brentwood
Essex CM13 1ZT
United Kingdom

http://www.chipmunkapublishing.com

Chipmunkapublishing gratefully acknowledges the support of Arts Council England.

Acknowledgements

I would like to dedicate this book to my two children Steven & Riana, who helped me find my inner strength and helped make it possible for me to write of my experience. Both children allowed me the opportunity to compare the differences in Autistic development together with typical development. To Steven who is Autistic helped me learn the true meaning of life where so much is taken for granted when all is going well. He let me absorb the strength in him while coping with his difficulties, while Riana who is a typical child, allowed me the opportunity to enjoy the expected rewards of a typically developing child. In addition she recognised the needs of her brother from an early age, where she learnt to stand by and offer a hand at every opportunity.

I would like to thank the National Autistic Society in acknowledging my story and putting me in contact with my publisher as well as for their continuous efforts in supporting all individuals with Autism and their families.

In addition I would like to acknowledge Dr Bernard Rimland (Founder of Autism Research Institute) through his work on the study and causes of Autism, Dr Ivor Lovaas in his approach to behavioural therapy, Temple Grandin PhD on her insider information on the Autistic persons perspective of the world, Leo Kanner in identifying the condition as a specific condition in recognising the associated traits, Hans Asperger in recognising a similar condition enabling the differentiation between the two diagnoses, Uta Frith on her books on the subject, Steven M.Edelson PhD (Centre for the Study of Autism, Salem, Oregon) for his research on the parts of the brain and its relationship to Autism, Mike Connor on his studies on Autism, S.F.T.A.H. (Society For the Autistically Handicapped) for their studies on the culture of Autism, Simon Baren-Cohen (Autism Research Centre) for his findings on the theory of mind, Catherine Maurice for the approach to behaviour intervention (ABA), Lorna Wing on her expert advice on the Autistic Spectrum Disorders and Donna Williams for sharing her courage in battling through the hardships of Autism.

NO MATTER WHAT

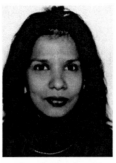

Biography of Sandy Howarth

Sandy was born in Colombo, Sri Lanka to Buddhist parents who were involved in a family owned furniture business. She was the youngest in a family of four children and attended an all girls school. She had a privileged lifestyle where she was completely isolated from any of life's hardships. Sandy is a descendent of the Anagarika Dharmapala who dedicated his life to spreading Buddhism throughout the world. She was a competitive swimmer and an artist and enjoyed every aspect of growing up in a tropical land.

Sandy worked in the family furniture factory prior to studying Art & Design at Derby Lonsdale College. The family business influence led her to further her studies in Interior Design at The Inchbald School of Design, London. Following her education in the UK she returned to Sri Lanka for a practical training year on a hotel project where she met her future husband. At the end of her training year she moved to New York to further her studies where she graduated with honours from Parsons School of Design. At the completion of her education she returned to Sri Lanka and got married later that year. Following her marriage she moved to London where she lived and worked for three years in hotel design and moved to Dubai for ten years.

Sandy continued her work in Interior Design in Dubai and spent some time in Oman during that time. In April 1994 her first child was born. She thought life was perfect until at two and a half years of age her son Steven was diagnosed Autistic. Her priorities changed where her life became Steven. She abandoned any thoughts of returning to work and decided to teach Steven instead. In March 1999 her daughter Riana was born.

Dubai didn't have any specialist teaching to help Steven and she decided in July 2000 to return to the UK. Having made many sacrifices to find what she hoped would be a good special needs school provision it soon became evident that his special educational needs were not being met. Following such a let down, she chose to withdraw Steven from the school and educate him at home following a strict home based programme which she delivered herself.

Sandy suffered health issues which took her energy away from focusing on Steven's education. Having suffered for three years she finally had her health sorted in August 2004 after which she felt that she had been given a new lease of life. She now feels that she has regained her energy to do what is best for Steven and the family.

Steven is now fifteen years old. After continuous struggles trying to obtain the best provision for Steven, Sandy has once again decided to teach Steven herself. She hopes that once Steven makes progress with his learning at home and when she is able to hire extra help to teach him that she will find time to pursue her passion for art and painting.

CONTENTS

- *Play in a manner that is unusual or odd*
- *Lack of awareness to danger*
- *Repetitive or obsessive behaviour*
- *Bizarre behaviour*
- *Hyperactive*
- *Passive*
- *Gives impression of being deaf or blind*
- *Spinning objects*
- *Laughing or crying for no apparent reason*
- *Prefer being alone*
- *Echolalia*
- *Lack of awareness of personal space*
- *Lack of facial expression*
- *Unusual body posture*
- *Lack of ability to imitate*
- *Lack of ability to sustain a conversation*
- *Lack of ability to gesture*
- *Poor eating habits*

11

with cognitive and communication disorders

53. **TYPES OF EDUCATIONAL PROVISION**
    (99-101)

- Mainstream school with a one-to-one classroom support
- Autistic unit attached to a mainstream school
- Mainstream school without one-to-one support
- Autistic school catering specifically for Autistic children
- Language unit catering for children with - language and communication difficulties
- Home based education

54. **METHODS USED IN TEACHING AUTISTIC CHILDREN (101-114)**

- *LOVAAS*
- *ABA (Applied Behaviour Analysis)*
- *PECS (Picture Exchange Communication System)*
- *TEACCH*

55. **SPEECH & LANGUAGE (104-107)**

56. *Typical speech & Language development*
57. *Speech & language problems in Autism*
58. *Encouraging speech development*
59. *Sign Language / Makaton*

60. **OCCUPATIONAL THERAPY** (107-110)
61. *Developing attention span*
62. *Developing sensory processing skills*
63. *Fine & Gross motor skills*
64. *Activities involving daily living*
65. *Visual perceptual skills*

66. ***Sensory Integration Therapy***
67. *Who would benefit from Sensory Integration Therapy?*

68. *Tactile defensiveness*
69. *Play Therapy*
70. *Holding Therapy*
71. *Dolphin Therapy*
72. *Option Therapy*
73. *Facilitated Communication*
74. *Physical Therapy*
75. *Computer Training*
76. *Vision Training - Irlene Lenses*
77. *Relationship development intervention*
78. *Social skills training*

79. **OTHER TREATMENTS** (114-119)

   - *Mega vitamin Therapy*
   - *Folic acid*
   - *Vitamin B6*
   - *Fish oil - EyeQ*
   - *Gluten - Casein free diet*
   - *Dimethyglycine supplements (DMG)*
   - *Secretin injection*
   - *Cranial Osteopathy*

What does the statement of educational needs contain?

- *Part 1 - Introduction of the child*
- *Part 2 - Special educational needs*
- *Part 3 - Special educational provision*
- *Part 4 - Placement*
- *Part 5 - Non Educational needs*
- *Part 6 - Non - Educational provision*

- All provision to be provided by the school or Authority or both
- Parental request for a statutory assessment

82. *Assessments*

83. *Who do you trust with assessments?*

84. **BATTLE FOR RIGHTS TO EDUCATION**
(132-142)

- *Attacks on Steven*
- *A result of a lack of choice*
- *Taking the LEA to Tribunal*
- *Reasons for pursuing tribunal proceedings - My child was placed in a provision that was inappropriate*
- *Procedures that followed*
- *What was included in the documentation*
- *Evidence of my child having regressed*
- *Evidence of attacks*
- *What steps did the LEA take?*
- *LEA's Defence*

- *Educational provision appropriate or inappropriate*

- *Dealing with Autistic behaviour - Distress : Understanding distress*
  Cause for distress
- *Confusion through having to accept a change in routine*
- *Confusion through change in teaching*
- *Frustration through having to wait or turn take*
- *Frustration through having to wait in a public setting*
- *Frustration through walking around a supermarket*
- *Distress through not being able to do as she/he wants*
- *Distress through confusion of departure*
- *Anger : Cause for anger*
  Result of anger
- *Anger through confusion in coping with the surrounding*
- *Anger through having to work*

- *Over excitement : Cause for over excitement*
  Result of over excitement
- *Hyperactivity through over excitement*
- *Rocking*
- *Flapping arms*
- *Attention seeking*
- *Obsessive behaviour*
- *Dealing with everyday situations*
- *Teaching your child to recognise rules*
- *Creating a bedtime routine*
- *Time out*
- *Redirecting negative behaviour*

- *Helping an Autistic individual to - understand and cope with their feelings*
- *Understanding and treating self - injurious behaviour*
- *Behaviour management rules*
- *How do Non Autistic peers see Autistic behaviour?*

89. **EARLY SIGNS OF BEHAVIOUR IN ("TYPICAL"/"AUTISTIC") DEVELOPMENT (181– 187)**

"Typical" development
- *Attachment, sharing interests or feelings*
- *Eye contact*

Autistic development
- *Lack of sharing interests and feelings*
- *Leading an adult by the hand*
- *Lack of imitation*
- *Lack of understanding the feelings of others*
- *Unusual language development*
- *Lack of attention*
- *Interaction with adults*

90. *Symptoms related to Autism*

- *Repetitive behaviour*
- *Resistance to change*
- *Self stimulory behaviour*
- *Head banging*

- *Will my child need care for the rest of his/her life?*
- *Will my child be accepted by society?*

101. **TEACHING LIFE SKILLS TO AUTISTIC CHILDREN (214-219)**

- *Learning to use the toilet*
- *Learning to wash hands*
- *Learning to dry hands*
- *Learning to wash face*
- *Learning to dry face*
- *Learning to brush teeth*
- *Rinsing mouth*
- *Washing hair*
- *Washing self*
- *Brushing hair*

102. **TEACHING BODY AWARENESS THROUGH PHYSICAL ACTIVITY (219-224)**

- *Using a swing*
- *Learning to hop*
- *Learning to throw / catch a ball*
- *Learning to kick a ball*
- *Learning to bounce a ball*
- *Learning to enjoy a roundabout / scooter*
- *Learning to ride a tricycle / bike*

Foreword

This has been written to enlighten the public of the immense struggles that individuals and families of Autism and related disorders are faced with. In explaining mental development Autism is observed alongside typical development to further demonstrate the bizarre nature of the condition. Research suggests that the human mind and nervous system remain plastic for a longer period than previously believed and that individuals with Autism are known to develop cognitively throughout their lives.

Autism is not an easy subject to explain to people as the Autistic thinking would seem almost incomprehensible to people who have not come into contact with an Autistic person. It takes time to understand it fully as it is a spectrum disorder where the individual with Autism could fit in anywhere within the spectrum.

This book offers support and guidance to families in recognising the expected challenges and suggests ways on how to help our children achieve their true potential. Advice is offered in dealing with typical day to day situations, dealing with education and developing skills, while gaining an insight into the subject of Autism.

In recognising a need to project awareness of Autism and it's complexities, I have explained the true meaning of Autism and included effective strategies used in coping and dealing with the condition.

Realising my son Steven's needs I taught myself the skills required to teach him. These included Speech &

Language Therapy, Physical Therapy, Play Therapy and Behaviour Therapy.

To manage Autism, learn to first accept Autism, think positively and act positively. Learn to love your child unconditionally, *'No matter what'* the diagnosis is. This is *your* child. A positive outlook will gain you the strength, to assist your child in every way. In recognising your acceptance your child will seek assurance from you, which will in turn help create a greater bond between you and your child.

Suggestions are offered to parent(s) who need to find time for themselves too. This will be a hard task at first which can be achieved through patience and perseverance. To bring about achieving any form of progress it is essential to make every obstacle a challenge and treat each step forward as a milestone. Your efforts will offer you the comfort of knowing that you have given your child a chance to reach their maximum potential. Autistic children vary in their behaviour, their level of intelligence and their ability to communicate. Nevertheless, they all fit into the broad Autistic spectrum and they all need help and support.

In the event that your child does not reach the level that you had expected, you can still be assured that you have done the best for your child. It is extremely difficult, almost impossible to predict the future of our children, but what you can do is to work on it now. *It is never too late*.

CHAPTER ONE

AUTISM - THE PUZZLING DISORDER

The word Autism derives from the Greek word *'auto'* which refers to self and directed from within. The condition is viewed as focusing on one's own interests and desires through an inability to focus beyond oneself. An unthinkably confusing and bizarre condition in which medical science desperately continues to search for answers with the hope of finding a cure in the not too distant future. The diagnosis of Autism shocks and terrifies the parents and families who feel that their worst nightmare has just come true. Starting with trauma, shame and denial, helplessness, guilt, blame, shattered hopes and broken marriages all become part of the process which impacts on the lives of the Autistic individuals and their families. Autism continues to be on the rise with little knowledge and much debate over its causes and puzzlement over the extremity in its effects.

The onset
Autism is a condition in which the disability is not easily recognised during the early stages of development. Though, in babies who display physical disabilities, a form of developmental disorder can be recognised from the time of birth. However, at times when there are no other disabilities present, two and a half years of age is a time to assess development in young children. Autism manifests between the times before birth to three years of age. Babies who have been different from birth are referred to as having

'early onset Autism' whilst others who have developed normally and shown signs of major regression indicate that these children had 'late onset regressive Autism'. Diagnosis often occurs during the toddler years, which leaves the parents to enjoy the baby years without any doubt that something could be wrong.

Detecting a difference before diagnosis
Parents may indicate concerns over their child being deaf due to a lack of response to the child's name or to commands being given to the child.

- A parent may be confused as to why their child walks away to be alone or avoids social interaction
- Behavioural oddities when comparing against a child's peer group
- The level of hyper-activity that keeps parents awake all day and all night will raise the question *"does my child never get tired?"*
- Adverse reaction to drugs and sedatives

Diagnosis
Parents of an Autistic child are faced with the long and stressful process of obtaining a diagnosis. Waiting for a diagnosis is an anxious time due to the uncertainty of what lies ahead. Dealing with day-to-day work and functioning normally is difficult when awaiting a diagnosis such as Autism, as the impact on your life is immense. Regardless, the recognition of the diagnosis is an essential part of the process which will assist in obtaining services and steering parents towards suitable treatment options.

Parents are faced with tiresome and endless demands. Coming to terms with the knowledge of Autism being a life long disability, dealing with the lack of public awareness of Autism, and attitudes towards Autism from friends and family are a few of the hurdles that parents are required to come to grips with.

A specialist will use a set of diagnostic standards to set Autism apart from other developmental disorders. Behaviour and ability are assessed according to what is typically expected of a child of the same age. Information will be gathered through observations of the child performing tasks, while taking note of the child's behaviours. On a non verbal level, intelligence is assessed through discussions with the parents, and through the child's ability to do puzzles and solve problems through everyday tasks.

For example, problem solving during the early stages of development was noted when Steven was first assessed at 2½ years of age. He spun and wrapped himself around the curtain in the paediatrician's consulting room. The paediatrician spun the curtain around and threw it over the pole to stop Steven from tearing the curtain down. Steven immediately observed the situation, found himself a chair to help him on to a bed in order to stand on the bed, and pull the curtain back down. This indicated a certain level of intelligence in finding a solution to achieve his goal.

Many specialists will hesitate to label a child Autistic until such time that they are absolutely certain of the diagnosis, as they do not want parents to lose hope. The specialist may use the general term P.D.D. (Pervasive Developmental Disorder) which appears less frightening to parents. No medical test or blood test can detect signs of Autism. On occasion children who show signs of slow learning, speech delay, hyper activity, lack of hearing, absent spells or poor vision may indicate traits of Autism.

The possibility of a diagnosis of Autism may lead to the specialist seeking further tests such as a hearing test, an eye test and, in instances where absent spells have been detected, an MRI scan. Such tests are not only distressing for the child but for the parents too. Autistic babies and children can demonstrate a great deal of physical strength when it comes to putting up resistance. Therefore it is wise to prepare yourself in as many ways as possible to help minimise the level of distress that the child is likely to experience. A test which can be carried out while the child is asleep should be performed during the child's sleep time. At times when it isn't practical to do so, a favourite toy can be used as a distracter. When there is no other alternative available, be prepared for a battle with the support of a few extra hands to help with the child.

Tests are carried out to alleviate and rule out the likelihood of complications related to hearing, vision, speech, and other neurological conditions. Once the tests have been completed and Autism appears to be implicated, the child will be referred to a specialist in Autism, who will conduct an assessment to determine the extent of the condition. The specialist will assess the information in precise detail and compare the results of the tests against other neurological conditions.

To be certain of an accurate diagnosis of Autism it is imperative to rule out other possible related mental conditions which indicate similar traits. A child who displays signs of mental retardation without the presence of Autistic traits will typically demonstrate an even level in all areas of development, while an Autistic child will indicate variability in development which, at times display extreme strength in one region and extreme weakness in another.

Furthermore, Autism is associated with an inconstancy in age expected development. The variability explains the reason behind the condition being recognised as a spectrum disorder where no two diagnoses are the same. In addition, the lack of uniformity in Autism has caused much confusion over the years leaving us guessing as to what to expect of the future of our children.

How parents feel
When starting a family a wish that is on every parents mind is that they have a healthy child. Parents do have doubts and thoughts of "what if their child has a disability," but for most it's only a passing thought. When the doubts are weighing heavy on an abnormality such as Down Syndrome, tests can be carried out through an amniocentesis. However, there are no pre-natal tests for Autism.

During the early years of parenting the behaviour of a

baby who is seen as difficult or placid may not be recognised as a cause for concern where it becomes accepted as a personality trait. Detecting a developmental disorder is particularly difficult in a first born child who looks physically healthy. An Autistic baby who doesn't suck well indicates early feeding problems. Such children may show a fascination with lights, dislike being held, swaddled or the process of nappy changing which all indicate signs of early sensory processing problems. For example Steven, as a newborn baby, indicated an extreme level of distress at being swaddled where he settled only to his swaddling cloth and his baby outfit being removed. In addition he demonstrated the same level of distress over the slightest wetness or soiling of his nappy.

MEDICAL TESTS

Medical tests are carried out to assist with the diagnosis and identify other related abnormalities.

Hearing test

An Audiogram and a Typanogram will detect if a child has a hearing impairment. The tests are done while measuring the responses when a sound is presented. The response indicated by turning a head or a blink of an eye at varying levels is able to determine any difficulties related to hearing.

EEG

Electroencephalogram - Brain waves are measured through an EEG which can detect signs of seizures, tumours or other abnormalities in the brain. Through this process of measuring electrical fields, an abnormally functioning brain will indicate a greater electrical potential to that of a normally functioning brain.

Metabolic screening

Blood and urine tests are carried out to determine the metabolic rate in food consumption in Autistic children to assess its effects on mental development. Tests that identify a nutritional deficiency will enable the nutrients which are lacking to be introduced into the diet of the Autistic child thereby, providing adequate nutrition to aid mental development. Dietary intervention has helped some Autistic children reduce their symptoms and make progress.

MRI

Magnetic Resonance Imaging - The use of magnetic sensing equipment creates a detailed image of the brain. During the scanning process the patient is expected to remain still in a long cylinder which is very noisy. A typical examination would take around thirty minutes. The image that is presented through the scan is similar to that of a CAT scan except it will show more detail in the soft tissues. MRI scans are most commonly used for patients who indicate seizure activity, spinal trauma and an unexpected loss of consciousness which is not a result of a stroke. The scan shows muscles, joints, bone marrow, blood vessels, nerves and structures within the brain and the body. The use of the scan is to examine the brain, the spine, the abdomen and the pelvis.

Although Steven has not shown signs of absent spells to date, I discussed Steven's family history of Epilepsy with his paediatrician. I wanted to know if there was a likelihood of Steven showing signs of seizure activity within his brain or the possibility of developing it later in life. I was alerted to what the scan entailed and the distress it could cause Steven. In addition, I was informed that even if the MRI scan was to detect an abnormality there may not be anything the medical world could do about it. It further confuses the issue, when researchers have noted size differences in certain regions of the brain in Autistic children but suggest that children with Autism do not have an abnormality that will show up on a MRI scan.

CAT SCAN

Computer Assisted Axial Tomography - An x-ray tube which rotates around the child and takes images of the brain and the body. The scanner was originally designed to take images of the brain though today it has advanced to take images of any part of the body. The scanner resembles a large doughnut which sends several beams simultaneously from different angles. The body of the patient is placed in the opening of the scanner and the bed moves backwards and forwards to allow the scanner to take the pictures. Each measurement made by the scanner is a cross section through the body/brain. CAT scans are useful in identifying structural abnormalities in the brain. The CAT scanner uses a lot more x-ray tubes than in ordinary x-rays, therefore doctors will only recommend its use with a good medical reason. The results show far more detail than in ordinary x-rays and the information received in two dimensional form can be used to reconstruct three dimensional images.

Confirmation of the diagnosis

The diagnosis of Autism will be confirmed when the child displays

- Limited or no eye contact
- Limited or no social awareness
- Limited or no communication
- Obsessive with routines
- Repetitive behaviour
- Fascination with spinning objects
- Aloofness

The diagnosis of Autism is crucial as it offers the parents an opportunity to learn of the necessary action to take. Standard methods of teaching cannot be applied to teaching children with Autism, therefore an accurate diagnosis enables parents to organise the provision that is most suited to meet the child's needs. Learning to recognise, understand and deal with the communication and social difficulties that are associated with Autism will help minimise the child's inbuilt frustrations in coping with the world.

Learning your child is Autistic

This is a tough challenge for any parent to accept. The lack of knowledge and awareness of the subject together with the uncertainties relating to the future, weigh heavily on the reluctance in accepting a condition such as Autism. Although, the term Autism is now widely known, the underlying impact is not well understood by the general public.

Parents and the families join in the joy of a new baby

and enjoy moments that may even be seen as stressful as part and parcel of parenthood. No parent would want to believe that something could be wrong with their child. When suspicions do arise, they look for reasons to dismiss those thoughts by gripping onto the belief that their child is perfect.

The disability takes a toll on your life and all aspirations you may have had for your child. The disability which is not evident at birth adds to the strain of accepting the condition, where parents are left confused, traumatised and helpless. Furthermore, it is an extremely tough undertaking for the specialist who conducts the assessment of the child, as they not only have to inform the parents of the child's condition but need to prepare themselves to deal with so much anger and disappointment from the parents as well. The messenger who delivers bad news is never welcome.

Dealing with the stress of the diagnosis
No parent expects to hear that their child is Autistic. In addition the shock of the diagnosis can leave parents drained of physical, mental and emotional energy. Therefore, it is important to conserve your energy to focus on areas of priority. Parents of Autistic children experience high stress levels, as everyday parenting skills are not adequate and effective when dealing with a child who is locked in their own little world.

The frustration, guilt, anger and resentment play a role in contributing to the added strain on the parents. Parents feel guilt as they blame themselves in feeling that perhaps the condition could have been avoided and frustrated in not being able to cope or get through to their child. Furthermore, a lack of external support adds to the difficulty in participating and enjoying everyday activities.

Allow others to support you in recognising the difficulties that you are faced with. This in turn will encourage those who genuinely want to assist, to offer support at times when coping becomes more than a challenge. Don't let yourself wallow in self pity, rather help yourself move through the process by recognising how you feel and find ways to deal with what you are experiencing. A friend who is ready to listen, or a diary in which you can write down and assess the process, will help you find a way forward.

Take care of yourself and look at relaxation methods to take your mind off the stressful situation. Give yourself time to accept your feelings and come to terms with the diagnosis. Seek professional help or counselling if you feel that you need it. Recognising your stress level is necessary in order to learn how to manage it. Following the diagnosis of Autism, parents are faced with fear, worry and anxiety which are the root causes of stress which results in an inability to cope. Excessive stress levels will lead to illness and stop you from doing the best for your child. A high stress level which leaves you mentally and physically exhausted on a regular basis means it is time to seek professional help.

The symptoms of stress can include a lack of sleep or insomnia, migraine headaches, loss of weight and gastritis. Your level of stress will lead to anxious and negative behaviour from your child. On the other hand learning to stay calm and focused will help you and the family cope effectively with a life changing diagnosis. A brighter outlook combined with methods of relaxation including yoga and breathing exercises, general physical fitness and a healthy diet will help you gain the energy to deal with the stress levels while moving forward towards a brighter future for all the family.

Parents need to recognise that Autism is long term when looking at effective methods of coping. Planning towards the future is the best way forward in dealing with an Autistic child.

Commitment level
Don't ever give up on your child saying it is hard work. *"It is hard work"* but your child needs you and above all your child must learn to live. Non-Autistic children learn a great deal from their peers, through sub-conscious observations to interpreting body language. All these areas need to be rote taught to Autistic children. Priorities should be aimed towards attaining life skills and social skills whereas the academic skills will follow in accordance with the level of ability.

What does the label mean?
In the vast majority of cases parents are said to be afraid of the label, which has been attributed to the fact that Autism is viewed as a no hope prognosis for their child. Some parents have expressed their thoughts in stating they felt they had received a life sentence.

There is both positive and negative in labelling an Autistic child. The positive being that an appropriate educational provision can be implemented in order to give the child the best possible chance in life. The child will be helped with minimising their frustrations and feel secure in an environment that understands their needs. On a negative note, to label a child who is only mildly Autistic, who is able to cope in a mainstream environment, might do more harm than good. A child who has developed language and has the potential to cope should be given the opportunity to cope and learn. Children do pick up habits from their peers and it is better that they pick up habits that are more socially accepted than not. Added specialist support in a mainstream setting would benefit children who are only mildly affected by Autism.

In addition, I believe that those children already labelled Autistic, who battle through the difficulties and learn to cope to the extent of leading normal lives, should be given a new label "Autism Defeated". This would help to remove the fear of the label and offer hope, strength and encouragement to parents knowing the difficulties are only minor and that much can be done to achieve their full potential. It would also add further pressure on the Education Authorities to aim towards achieving that label thereby, creating a happier group of people.

Creating public awareness
An invisible condition such as Autism creates further barriers towards developing public awareness of what the condition is about. Despite the publicity gained

through the MMR debate which has given a wider knowledge of the term, most people do not have a clue about the wider picture and what the parents or carers are experiencing.

Being disgruntled at the public for a lack of awareness of a disability which is clearly not visible isn't fair. You may experience a lack of sympathy, certainly a lack of empathy and will almost certainly be subject to comments that are hurtful.

I believe in taking steps to prevent any setbacks in social situations. However, at times when it isn't possible to prevent a situation, it will be easier to give out a card which reads:

Please don't let my child's behaviour disturb you. My child is Autistic. Autism is: A neurological disorder in which the individual lives in a world of their own. The behaviour is a result of a lack of understanding of social rules.
For further information contact: The National Autistic Society

Alternatively cards carrying a similar message can be obtained from the National Autistic Society.

In this situation you can pass on the message in a fast and effective way. You could also try explaining to people about your child's Autism which will require a bit more of your time, but either way you have got the message across which will spread a little more understanding on the subject of Autism. This is a positive approach which will receive a positive reaction.

Help for parents
It is an absolute must that parents receive the help that they deserve. Parents need to gain sufficient energy to enable them to cope with the Autistic child as well as coping with the rest of the family. The most effective way to introduce your Autistic child to expectations within the home environment is to recognise the demands placed on the family alongside the needs of the rest of the family. Therefore, a clear identification of the individual needs within the family will help put things in place for the complete family. Friends and relatives could do their bit in offering emotional and mental support though, that sometimes is not forth coming. Autistic children display challenging behaviour which can be very stressful; therefore, engaging more people who are experienced in dealing with your child will lend a hand in ensuring an easier life for you, your child and the family.

Autistic family life
Raising children is a strain on most parents as each family copes with their responsibilities based on their experience, knowledge and ability to cope. As the saying goes "the stresses and joys of parenthood". Parents learn to understand the personalities of each child and their children learn to recognise the personalities of their parents and other family members.

Coping in an environment which clearly lacks the acceptance of Autism, a lack of social support and dealing with an Autistic child's antisocial behaviour are a few of the challenges that parents are faced with. In addition it has been noted that an Autistic child manifests existing problems within a family or for others creates new areas of conflict.

When living with an Autistic child the stresses are so much greater than in a non-Autistic household, as the Autistic child has problems in not only relating to other people but recognising that others have needs too. Some of the challenges in living with Autism could be sleep disorders, a lack of understanding in relating to others, barriers in communication, a lack of ability to care for themselves, and food and sensory intolerances. As a result Autism impacts on the lives of the rest of the family.

The lack of ability to communicate while making sense of the world is the greatest barrier to an individual with Autism. Events which most people accept as normal everyday situations could cause a great deal of anxiety or fear to an Autistic child.

Most individuals with Autism have added learning disabilities and some suffer from Epilepsy. The added difficulties add more pressure on families coping with the disability. The difficulties outlined, not only cause an enormous strain on the family, but also leave them feeling isolated. Some express sadness, anger and resentment. Some parents find it too much to cope with the added pressure resulting in the break-up of marriages. Some find it difficult to cope emotionally and mentally and often suffer depression. The stresses have been brought to public attention as a result of some high profile incidents that have been reported in the past years, such as murder/suicide of Autistic children and their prime carers. All families require as much support and guidance to deal with their unexpected challenges and enable them to lead happier lives.

It has been reported that the divorce rate in families with an Autistic child is around 80%. Dealing with the stress of the diagnosis, behavioural issues, lack of trained staff, lack of support from services, social issues, financial stress to provide adequate long term support are but a few of the factors that add to the stress of any marriage.

In families with an Autistic child, it tends to be the case that one parent stays remote from the situation and the other gets over involved, typically the dad focuses on his work and the mum focuses on the needs of the Autistic child. This doesn't leave any room for shared interests which leaves the couple moving in separate directions. Therefore, keeping the lines of communication open means that you can do more to help your child. It is most desirable that parents share the responsibility 50-50, but the chances of this happening are remote. For the sake of the family and the partnership the parent who is most involved needs to have scheduled breaks in order to cope effectively. Some parents run away from their responsibilities, their marriage and even their Autistic child.

Look at respite services available and if you have the

finances available you can hire trained people to provide the care that your child needs. Avoiding burnout is an essential part of being a good parent for an Autistic child and shows that you are in control and have effective coping strategies in place.

Mothers of Autistic children are said to suffer a great deal of emotional trauma, as they often hold themselves responsible for their child's behaviour. Fathers of Autistic children are less affected as they tend to suppress their feelings, whereas mothers vent their feelings by going through a range of grieving processes.

I believe that Autism is a strength. Taking note of the neurotypically wired majority of the human race, how many would be able to comprehend living in an Autistic world? The Autistic child did not ask to be Autistic. It is confusing, it is bizarre, it is scary, and it is lonely just to outline a few scenarios in the mind of an Autistic person. They need the support of all humankind to learn to understand them. Like all people, Autistic individuals also have their own limitations but they most certainly have their own strengths. Given the best chance to realise their potential they are capable of being the best they can.

"Living with Autism is a challenge to most families, but living in our world is a greater challenge to an individual with Autism. Help them in their journey through life."

Understanding self

An individual self is made up of sensations, emotions, thoughts and perception. Information from these areas is gathered, processed and presented to our conscious and sub-conscious being. The connection between these areas links the self together which allows us to function as individual beings. An absence of these connections would make it impossible for the self to function, which would mean that the self is asleep. The 'I' function which relates to self is lacking or works differently in the Autistic person. They do have thoughts while some do experience self reflections but in most situations the Autistic individual has to be taught to recognise themselves.

The connectivity in the brain of an Autistic individual shows irregularities where the conscious being is awake in some regions and asleep in other regions. This explains an imbalanced function which results in an imbalanced life through a distorted inner self.

Understanding the theory of self will help in learning to interact with the Autistic and non Autistic self and help bring the two closer together.

The fear of the unknown

Many Autistic behaviours arise not only from an underdeveloped nervous system, under sensitive or oversensitive senses but from the fear of the unknown. This fear stems from a lack of awareness of what the world around them means. A fear which is not only related to an Autistic individual but to most human behaviour. The non-Autistic population that cannot comprehend the bizarre symptoms associated with Autistic behaviour will express a certain level of caution when approaching an Autistic individual, or will avoid approaching the individual altogether. To reject an Autistic child with an inbuilt social and communication disorder will not help them; rather it will further isolate them from society pushing them to further withdraw into themselves. Accept them and they will accept living in our world. This is the only way to bring the Autistic and non Autistic worlds together.

The beauty of innocence

In days gone by, when the existence of Autism was not known it was believed that the angels had taken away their baby and left an angel baby in its place. Autistic babies and children do look angelically beautiful. For example, at the time of Steven's birth in Dubai, I had other new mums walking over to get a glimpse of my baby and the comment, "what a beautiful baby" was often made. Steven entered this world lacking any creases and appeared so perfectly fresh and there was a distinct difference in Steven as compared with other babies. It turned out all too good to be true when I returned home with him and he cried all night, I thought there was something more seriously wrong as I just could not find a way to console him.

Having observed other Autistic children and teenagers, I believe that a major part of the beauty lies in their eyes which look vacant and innocent and lacking in the ability to manipulate in a typical sense. Their beauty is enhanced to a greater extent as they don't understand vanity or the meaning of being beautiful. Their needs are simple and based on survival mechanisms to cope in a complex world which most take for granted.

Feeling alone and rejected

Feeling alone is something that most parents experience. All parents of Autistic children must learn that they are not alone. Every parent of an Autistic child has been through the same concerns which are all natural reactions from any caring parent. Rejection is hard to deal with but, as a parent, if you are rejected because of your child, don't let it affect you, just focus on your child.

Going into denial

At times when the diagnosis of the Autism is too much to contend with, parents go into denial. This is a reaction which many parents experience, where no amount of counselling will alter the situation with your child. Invariably, the parents need to come to terms with the Autism themselves to help their child and look towards a future for their child. Another vital factor for both parents is to support each other emotionally. It isn't only parents who go into denial, but relatives and friends find it difficult to accept too. Therefore, the sooner the parents accept the Autism the sooner all others will, and the sooner the real work of helping the child can begin.

Dealing with an Autistic child after the initial diagnosis

A carer who lacks experience will find it difficult to deal with a child with Autism, but anyone with a genuine will both to learn and to take up the challenge can gain the required skills. Do not be upset by Autistic behaviours but look at ways of dealing with behaviours, whilst minimising and eliminating them if they are seen as unacceptable. At times when an Autistic child does not seek your affection do not feel rejected, but offer it to the child anyway. Offering affection to your child will aid your child in feeling secure where they will show a need for that security. Look at it from their perspective, how it must feel to be locked away unable to communicate with the rest of the world. Therefore, support your child in finding ways to help them out of their world and into our world.

WHAT DOES AUTISM MEAN?

Autism was first recognised by Leo Kanner in 1943. Following the recognition, Hans Asperger in 1944 identified a condition which had similar traits to Autism which is known today as Asperger's Syndrome. There are a great number of text books defining Autism and what it means, both in academic and real terms. I have included as many of the challenges a person with Autism is faced with in explaining the condition. Autism means that an individual displaying Autistic traits has difficulty in the areas of communication, social and emotional development and imagination. They appear to be indifferent and aloof living in a world of their own, where they are unable to form emotional bonds and lack the understanding, thoughts and feelings of others.

- *Difficulty with verbal communication*
Many Autistic individuals display difficulty using language to communicate. The world is all about communication and interaction with people. An Autistic child, who does not acquire meaningful language or learn to use gestures, cannot communicate their needs. Often, Autistic children who do develop language understand language in a literal sense making phrases, idioms and metaphors incomprehensible to them.

- *Difficulty with non-verbal communication*
Many Autistic children display difficulty using gestures to communicate. During typical development children who lack language skills will point, nod or shake their heads to communicate but the Autistic individual shows a lack of awareness of the use of gestures to compensate for their absence in speech development.

- *Lacking in social development*
Many Autistic children display difficulty in absorbing stimulation from the environment. Typical children with no language skills will learn social play through watching and observing others but the Autistic child cannot comprehend the meaning of social play. The inability to recognise a need for social interaction results in an Autistic individual avoiding social situations.

- *Lacking in emotional development*
Many Autistic children and adults experience difficulties in expressing their emotions as well as

understanding and reading the emotions of others. This difficulty causes frustration and can result in inappropriate behaviour.

- ***Lacking in imagination***
Most Autistic children display difficulty with imaginative play, compared with "typical" children who enjoy this stage of development where they do not need any encouragement to imitate their parents or what appears on TV. As children grow up the imitation takes a more advanced role where it leads to imagination. Autistic children who do not imitate others or use pretend play, can however demonstrate a level of creativity in one area of interest where most of their thoughts are concentrated just in that one area.

- ***Lacking or no eye contact***
A recognisable early sign of Autism where the child makes a conscious effort to avoid eye contact. This tendency results from a lack of social need where the child would take an adult by the hand to get what they want rather than use eye contact to share interest or communicate. Some Autistic children do use eye contact though it is not as regular and spontaneous and unusual or different to non Autistic children.

- ***Insistence on routine***
The world is a bizarre place to an Autistic child. They need a great deal of support to feel secure in their environment. They crave for routine to help maintain some form of stability in their otherwise confused world. I believe that it is necessary to help the Autistic child develop through a routine and a structured day.

However, introducing changes will teach flexibility to an Autistic child in learning to adjust and accept living in our world.

- *Difficulty with taking turns*

Most Autistic behaviour stems from a frustration which has risen through a lack of awareness of the world we live in. An Autistic child sees the world and only their immediate needs where they demonstrate a lack of awareness of the needs of others. As a result waiting and turn taking can be quite frustrating for the Autistic child who doesn't understand social rules.

- *Over or under sensitive senses*

A child who is overly sensitive to touch will hold themselves rigidly and reject a hug. A child who has over sensitive hearing will express difficulty in coping with everyday sounds. For example, the sound of a washing machine or vacuum cleaner or extreme temperatures could cause a great deal of distress to some children while others may not react at all.

- *Play in a manner that is unusual or odd*

The lack of imagination in Autistic children restricts their ability to play in a way that is typical. They tend to play in a manner that is obsessive or repetitive and could get fixated on one thing such as the wheels on a car.

- *Lack of awareness of danger*

The inability to understand our world means they could wander off being completely oblivious to danger as well as not have a concept of road safety or a fear of heights.

- ***Repetitive or obsessive behaviour***
Lacking in imagination and the inability to be flexible with their thoughts results in repetition in their behaviour.

- ***Bizarre behaviour***
Commonly this involves flapping arms, moving fingers in front of their eyes, head banging, rocking and walking on tiptoes.

- ***Hyperactive***
Many Autistic children tend to be hyperactive and at times the effort to tire them out seems endless. The difficulty in sleeping is the brain's inability to switch off, which becomes a vicious cycle. Some hyperactive children react to additives and food colourings.

- ***Passive***
A lack of awareness of social rules or what is expected in terms of willing participation will indicate passive behaviour in an Autistic child. For example, a child who accepts any role that others foist upon them, rather than argue and express their preference.

- ***Gives impression of being deaf or blind***
Some do not react to certain environmental sounds or show an awareness of the presence of others.

- ***Spinning objects***
Some Autistic children are overly stimulated by spinning or things that spin.

- *Laughing or crying for no apparent reason*

Autistic children show difficulty in recognising or processing their own emotions which results in laughing or crying for different reasons.

- *Prefer being alone*

An Autistic child may wander off to be on their own or reject being in a room full of people. This is a result of a lack of interest in others which is apparent from a very early age.

- *Echolalia*

The child repeats or parrots words or phrases due to an inability to comprehend what has been heard. Some children with Autism can memorise and repeat complete phrases. I heard the term "echolalia" when Steven was first diagnosed with Autism. I was rather alarmed to learn that echolalia meant meaningless language, and I recall having nightmares over it. However, as time went on and it became apparent that spontaneous language wasn't coming forth so easily, I hoped and waited for Steven to begin using echolalia knowing that it would be a start. I reassured myself, thinking that once Steven started using echolalia I could help him put it into place.

- *Lack of awareness of personal space*

Starting with eye contact where they feel uneasy at first but once they have learnt to use it they use it with carers or family or in a manner that is odd. Some Autistic children feel threatened by touch, or by the invasion of personal space when being stood next to or in the same room that the child is in. On the other hand some who do use regular eye contact may stand very close and stare. This explains though some Autistic children understand their own space by withdrawing to be alone that some don't understand the needs of others when invading the space of others.

- ***Lack of facial expression***
The lack of awareness of their own thoughts and feelings will result in a lack of facial expression in an Autistic individual.

- ***Unusual body posture***
The lack of awareness of themselves and their own body results in an unusual body posture.

- ***Lack of ability to imitate***
Autistic children show a lack of interest in observing others. They do not connect the behaviour of other people to themselves which makes it difficult to imitate others.

- ***Lack of ability to sustain a conversation***
A lack of interest in others will lead to a conversation which is self directed or used as a means to serve a need.

- ***Lack of ability to gesture***
Autistic children lack the understanding of non verbal communication which results in helping themselves or reaching for what they want, rather than pointing to communicate a need.

• *Poor eating habits*
Children with Autism tend to demonstrate restricted eating habits where their interest in food is limited or nonexistent.

In further explaining the difficulties associated with Autism it must be noted that as typical human beings our brains are wired in a way which allows us to absorb and adapt to new information, while altering our thinking to suit a particular situation. We learn through every situation. Our conscious and subconscious minds work together, allowing us to take in information, store, reason, challenge and conclude upon our decisions. The decisions we make are based on a process of thoughts. In addition, we build on previously gained knowledge and feel secure in reinforcing that knowledge.

Autistic individuals, though they may not all exhibit vision or auditory impairments, show signs of sensory processing difficulties when exposed to the world around them. As a result they feel overwhelmed by what they see, hear or feel.

An Autistic child could act in a similar manner to a deaf or blind child when they walk into things, look past people, depend on holding an adults hand to be led and do not respond to environmental sounds or being spoken to. Most people with normal vision rely 80% on their ability to see in obtaining information from the environment. In contrast a blind child lives his world 100% in darkness, where he/she has to use all of the other senses to compensate for the lack of vision to be able to make sense of the world. Here the blind child has a clear physical reason for having difficulty processing information through visual means. An Autistic child's inability to process information from the environment is a result of the neurological complexity of the condition which makes it difficult to integrate their senses.

In addition an Autistic individual experiences difficulties in using language effectively. This barrier is caused by a lack of the inbuilt mechanism that processes and creates the structure of language.

Recognising sensory sensitivities in Autistic children
Sensory sensitivities vary in most Autistic individuals. An Autistic individual who covers their ears to the sound of a loud noise indicates a sign of hearing sensitivity. Extreme sensitivity will be demonstrated by a child showing distress associated with a loud noise. Children with visual and auditory sensitivity could indicate normal hearing and vision through tests carried out, which can leave specialists rather confused. Further confusion is caused as some Autistic individuals find sharp sounds or bright lights unbearably painful, whereas some enjoy them and others do not react to them.

Steven displayed signs of mild hearing sensitivity starting from his toddler years to the age of four years. It was evident at the time as he covered his ears to sounds made by certain electronic devices. During this time an AIT (Auditory Integration Training) specialist from the UK arrived in Dubai. This was the early stages of the diagnosis when I was desperate to try anything to help Steven.

Steven was four years of age when he received a ten day programme of AIT. The first four days of the training was challenging as Steven was extremely distressed with having to wear headphones to listen to sounds that seemed to be causing him distress. However, with the hope of it benefiting Steven, I persevered. Steven learnt to relax on the fifth day and by the sixth day accepted and went on to enjoy the sounds that he was listening to. This was the start of his interest in music and he now listens to a variety of music in addition to calming himself to music. He has shown an interest in classical, pop, opera, piano and the music of Disney. Although, Steven will cover his ears on occasion, it is now associated with confusion caused by an unexpected situation. An action which is sometimes associated with stopping in his tracks accompanied by a smile indicates it as his way of coping with the sudden pleasant change. Although this is a positive experience for Steven, I help him put his hands down and hold his hands to offer him the reassurance that he is looking for.

CHAPTER TWO

MIND BLINDNESS, INNOCENCE & GRATITUDE

Thinking in Autism

Understanding the way an Autistic child thinks is necessary when choosing an effective method of teaching. Autistic thoughts which are not communicated using normal modes of expression, cause confusion to the person who is trying to read and understand those thoughts. However, taking the time to feel and experience their thinking is a valuable way forward in aiding them through their areas of difficulty.

Autistic children have the potential to learn. However, at times when that potential is not recognised and the necessary support is not provided they may be trapped in a world that is confusing and incomprehensible to them for a very long time. Some children are able to show signs of exceptional skills from an early age where they gain the ability to further their potential starting from early on in life. However, children who display difficulty in recognising their own strengths are more difficult to assess and they lose out on maximising their true potential. Once strengths and weaknesses are assessed accurately an emphasis should be placed on further enhancing the strengths whilst developing those areas of weakness. Every parent must play a role in enriching their child's future.

Many strengths develop through interests. Therefore, a great deal of emphasis needs to be placed on the recognition of a particular interest, in order to observe and work towards the child's true potential. Recognising an interest is beneficial in further encouraging learning through developing thinking skills too. It is said that highly intelligent people are very good at solving puzzles or mathematical problems where they have the pieces required to solve the puzzles but that they are not so good when it comes to finding the answers through assessing and processing the missing links themselves. An area that many Autistic individuals struggle with is the ability to understand, process and find a solution.

With support for some and a great deal of input for others Autistic children can be taught to think. It has been said to have been left too late where it turns out to be more difficult to deal with the child or the symptoms associated with Autism. I believe that it is never too late. Once the areas of difficulty have been recognised, a great deal of commitment in delivering the required level of help will help your child progress. Tasks which are made easy and fun to start with will motivate learning while developing thinking skills, as a child who enjoys an activity is more likely to develop the required skill.

Theory of mind
Starting from the age of two-three years, neuro-typical children learn the theory that other people have minds too. This aspect is lacking in socially impaired children. Although two-three years is the onset at which time theory of mind develops it is possible to recognise signs from a very early age. When observing a baby, or a

very young child, the lack of eye contact to communicate, the rigidity when held and a general disinterest in people, is a clear sign of an anti social disorder, which in turn indicates the lack of theory of mind.

An Autistic child whose thinking is obscure results in a difficulty in using their own thinking as a model. In turn it causes a lack of awareness in understanding the intents of others. Simon Baron Cohen explains that for an individual to have a theory of mind mechanism, they must have the shared attention mechanism which is displayed when two people focus their attention on the same object. He describes mind reading as the "capacity to imagine or represent states of mind that we or others hold" and states that "mind reading is enabled by the language faculty". He further supports his theory that the ability to mind read develops before the development of language by stating that the mind reading system, unless wired to the language faculty which allows us to inform, exchange and question would not be made possible. The language will be used in a concrete manner rather than in a social sense. His theory further supports the complexity of the Autistic brain which trains the Autistic individual to think in a concrete sense where they lack the flexibility of thought.

Humour & Autism
Humour is the most effective way of enriching the life of an Autistic individual as well as helping to lighten the load on the lives of their parents and carers. Just as most people, who look at Autistic behaviour, think it is

odd and therefore it is funny, the Autistic person could look at non-Autistic behaviour and think it funny too. The world we live in interprets anything that's not standard as being odd. A behaviour, which does not affect the persons development in achieving skills or doesn't upset others, could be something that the Autistic individual is given time to enjoy. As humour is based on what contradicts our usual social understanding, the idea that most Autistic people don't hold the same social understanding means that something that is seen as humorous to the rest of us may be lost on an Autistic person.

Apportioning blame

This is a first reaction from many parents. The inability to deal with such a life changing situation leaves most parents looking to escape from accepting the cause for their child's condition. However, when dealing with experts it is vital that questions are answered as accurately as possible with a view to helping your child as well as offering support towards research and findings. The blame stems from the total lack of understanding and acceptance of Autism. Autism is a puzzle. The first reactions are *"how could it be possible for a perfectly healthy looking baby to suddenly become Autistic?"* This is an extremely hard and painful concept to accept. However, if your love for your child is unconditional, you will find it easy to accept and deal with the obstacles and thereby, offer your child the best possible chance in life.

Is it the MMR vaccine?
My child regressed after the MMR vaccine at 15 months just as a large proportion of other Autistic children did. I do not blame the vaccine for Steven's Autism, as having studied Steven very closely I recognised that he displayed behaviour that was different or lacking in normal development even before the time when the regression took place. I had concerns over Steven's level of activity, his erratic sleep pattern and the comprehension of language before he had his MMR vaccination. I was only able to learn this by studying Steven very closely. I had taken Steven to a baby group from the age of 4 months, thereafter to a toddler group where I was constantly observing Steven alongside other babies and toddlers. Furthermore, Steven and I travelled for 2 months during the time of the vaccination. In my view, although Steven seemed to develop many age appropriate skills by the time he reached 15 months, he did not possess enough to be called non-Autistic. 15 months is an age where most toddlers assert themselves and become aware of themselves. If the Autism was lying dormant in his system this could have been a time that it triggered.

Recognising Steven's loss of skills after the MMR vaccination together with symptoms in behaviour before the MMR could have meant a genetic susceptibility which triggered at a certain age in his development. I cannot say if the MMR acted as a trigger and enhanced the severity of the Autism or if it was caused by some other environmental factor or even just the age where he recognised his own difficulties. Whatever the reason, I had to look at ways of helping

Steven learn to cope with the world. However, I did not hesitate to give Steven's younger sister the vaccination when it was due, as I was clear from her level of alertness that Autism was not a factor.

Whatever the reason

It is negative to apportion blame. If the results of surveys carried out means it will get to the cause and help prevent Autism, that is positive but for now we need to deal with the condition and being positive will give you a good start.

Dealing with siblings

Siblings are special too. Due to the huge demands an Autistic child places on a family, siblings tend to feel left out. It is natural for siblings to feel left out. Therefore, the siblings need to be taught a little bit about Autism and ways to deal with it, as well as be included in any play and turn taking activities. The Autistic child should also be made to follow the same rules that apply to the rest of the children, and siblings should be rewarded equally for good work as well as for helping their Autistic brother/sister. This would result in the sibling feeling accepted and willing to help. Families will benefit from an Autistic child having more than one sibling due to the added support to share the load. A sibling of an Autistic child takes on an adult role very early on in life where it is particularly so if there isn't another adult present at home.

Love and discipline

As with all children Autistic children need love as well as discipline. Offering love to your Autistic child should offer comfort to you as well as your child. Some Autistic children may reject comfort but once you have passed the barrier, it will be a major step towards your child's happiness and feeling of acceptance. You could start with a gentle touch to a hug. However, if your child will not tolerate physical contact you could try other ways to make a connection. For example, give me five or shaking hands or even link fingers.

Just as much as love and reassurance is important, discipline is as important. Just as many children do, an Autistic child will push boundaries as far as they can. Here a strict and consistent approach is necessary in order to assist the Autistic child to understand and comply with the rules that have been set.

WHAT DOES THE AUTISTIC CHILD TEACH YOU?

- *Patience*

What takes place naturally in normal development will be very slow in an Autistic child. Everything needs to be taught. Life becomes a constant waiting game.

- *Looks can be deceptive*

Since it is not always visible at first sight Autism will often baffle people.

- *Honesty and innocence*

An Autistic child is innocent and needs more than a helping hand to learn to cope with the world around them.

- ***To give love unconditionally***

An Autistic child will only learn to understand love if you offer love without any expectations. The joys that a parent receives from having a normally developing child are not present in an Autistic child but there are different joys which cannot be expressed.

- ***To be grateful for small mercies***

Love the child you have and treat each step forward as a milestone

- ***To be understanding of others in distress***

Words cannot describe the immense trauma that parents are faced with in having an Autistic child. Coming to terms and learning to cope is a part of the healing process, which helps you understand how others in distress must feel.

- ***To focus on priorities***

An Autistic child changes your life to a degree where you find a balance to focus on what is truly important and ignore petty details.

- ***To find the strength and energy to do things you never thought possible***

An Autistic child will push boundaries way beyond that of a normally developing child. The parent needs to be constantly tuned in to predict and act on unexpected behaviours or situations.

- ***To sharpen your sense of awareness***

Autistic behaviours keep parents constantly listening or looking out for what the child is up to.

Will the Autism ever go away?

Autism is a life long mental impairment that medical science has yet to learn of a complete cure to treat it.

Methods of treatment have been tried and tested, but these methods do not always work for every child. In desperation parents will try every method of treatment that is within their reach. These methods make it not only a waiting game, but also a guessing game. ***What is most important is to give priority to education.***

Parents' views

Most parents have strong and different views on the treatments and approaches used in Autism. They are behavioural interventions, dietary treatments, cognitive therapies and medications. Teachers who work with Autistic children vary greatly in their strengths, their ability to deal with Autism and their ability to deal with the constant challenges faced with a lack of available resources. Students on the Autistic spectrum vary in their ability to function in an educational environment or deal with everyday functions. Therefore, the amount of support required has to be determined by the level of functioning in each individual. Teachers are well aware of the need, but the limited resources available means that the Autistic child may not receive the required method of treatment that he/she needs. A major factor associated with allocating resources is down to the authorities who are responsible for making the resources available. They lack the first hand experience with the true challenges faced by individuals with Autism. Although it is widely acknowledged that parents of Autistic children are far more knowledgeable in advising staff of effective methods to meet their child's needs, this knowledge is frequently ignored.

Parent's want their children to fit in. A child who

doesn't fit in to any environment is seen as a problem. It's not just Autism, but in any situation if you don't fit in you are isolated from the rest. As human beings we are social creatures and an anti social disorder such as Autism creates a barrier with not just family but society as a whole. The difficulty with Autism is not only that the Autistic child refuses to participate in activities that the rest of the family enjoy, but that they do not have any concept of what the activity means. Therefore, help them in learning to enjoy and participate in activities which take their interest.

CHAPTER THREE

STEVEN'S DEVELOPMENTAL HISTORY
LEARNING THE HARD FACTS

Steven is my first-born child. He was born in Dubai at 37 weeks gestation weighing 3.55kg. Healthy at birth, Steven was extremely demanding for the first 10 weeks of his life, as he suffered from colic. Once the colic had passed he was active, happy and sociable for the most part. Steven sat at 6 months, crawled at 7½ months, ran on tiptoes at 10½ months and was climbing stairs at 13 months. Steven smiled at 4 weeks, blew kisses and waved bye-bye appropriately at 10 months. At the age of 1 year he imitated cleaning and throwing specs of dirt in the bin, he enjoyed picking up the phone to the sound of the ring and responded appropriately by saying "hello," hid under the table or cot to be found and toppled building blocks. He rode a toy truck from one year onwards pushing it along with his feet. Steven's favourite interest from the age of one year has been Disney videos. He had approximately five words at 10 months and these words were used in context, though, they tended to disappear by the age of 16 months.

Recognising early signs of Autism in Steven
Having been to antenatal classes and not had any reason to believe that anything could be wrong with my baby, I looked forward to the birth of my new baby. I learnt as much as I needed to learn about babies and what comforted them and how they responded, together

with what was expected at each stage of development. One of my early thoughts was how I was to hold my baby soon after it was born, to allow the baby to recognise me and start the bonding process. When Steven was born, I found the holding process a little odd, as I held Steven and he lay there not looking at me. I had learnt that babies enjoyed being held close but my baby wanted to feel free. The feeding pattern too was different as he didn't seem to enjoy the typical feeding ways, when held close to me and at times, when he was held close, he didn't make the expected eye contact. Once Steven went onto solids at sixteen weeks, although he did eat pureed food, I could never be certain of which foods he preferred, as there was a lack of expression or signs of eagerness in looking forward to his meal or any expression of having enjoyed his food. There was very little communication and interaction was mostly associated with rough and tumble play or to serve a need.

I had bought a baby book by Anne Geddis when my baby was born which I looked forward to filling in. I found the book interesting and realised that the questions posed in the book relating to interests and behaviour would give early pointers to my child's personality starting from a very young age. It became clear that, as Steven grew, I could not answer many of the questions as these related to early developmental mile stones and did not correspond with Steven's progress or interests. In addition, his lack of expression made it all a guessing game to know of his preferences during the early years.

Interaction with others

Steven was taken to a weekly baby group from the age of 4 months where he seemed very much the same as other babies. However, once he moved on to a toddler group the first signs of "difference" became apparent. During this time he was extremely hyperactive. He could not stay still for even a second. Despite a tendency to be overactive, he enjoyed playing with toys, where he did so appropriately, while being comfortable around other children. Steven was seen as the clumsy toddler who constantly fell into the toy box. Where other toddlers would express their wants through sounds or words Steven was determined to fetch his toy himself. Reflecting on Steven's early years, the recurrence of self reliant behaviour indicated a lack of social and communication awareness from an early age.

As time went on, when Steven approached his toddler years, he started withdrawing himself, preferring to be on his own. I found children in general to be unassuming, where they were ready to make friends in play as well as social situations. However, things didn't quite add up with Steven. Children of two to three years of age would approach Steven and ask him his name and he would ignore them. At this age, it was easy to explain to a two a young toddler by saying "Steven doesn't talk." Some would approach him without language but would still find ways to interact through babbling, or eye contact, while constantly showing interest in doing so.

My observations of Steven with his peer group were in Dubai at a swimming club when children made an effort to interact with him. They would keep attempting to interact and finally give up or interact with Steven via myself who helped him learn and participate in activities which he had resisted to start off with.

Steven had to be constantly watched not just for his lack of awareness, but to stop him from upsetting others. For instance, he would walk up to a child and try to lick the child's ice-lolly while the child was holding onto it. The child holding the ice-lolly would look so confused as he pulled his hand away and found that Steven had no interest in looking at the child to communicate an interest in the ice-lolly, all he was interested in was to help himself to the ice-lolly. Steven indicated a total lack of awareness of the needs of others or the presence of others.

Early Travel
Steven had his first trip abroad at 7½ months. He travelled to England where we had a base, New Zealand to visit his father's family and to Sri Lanka where my family live. Steven coped well with the travelling and enjoyed Christmas in England where he joined in the festive activities. He thoroughly enjoyed the outdoor space in New Zealand and the beaches in Sri Lanka.

Can grandmas cope? An incident in New Zealand
Grandma was asked to baby sit Steven one evening and was given instructions on how to deal with Steven. Steven was around 8 months of age at this time and he was extremely attached to me. On our return we found Steven fast asleep in his travel cot, his hair soaking wet

and grandma seated awake, also with soaking, wet hair. The wet hair indicated that both Steven and grandma had suffered a great deal of distress together with a physical workout. Knowing from the look on grandma's face and what she would have gone through, I comforted her.

Grandma's response

"I gave the soother like you said, he spat it out."

"I gave the juice like you said; he threw the darn thing away."

"I carried him and rocked him like you said. Oh no! He didn't want that."

"Anyway I'm still alive."

Having not been aware of Steven's Autism at the time I can now look back on how his extreme dependency on me led to challenging behaviour, even as an infant. It didn't ease at the age of three to four years when other children were able to trust more than just the immediate parents to attend to their needs. In recognising the level of dependency from an early age, my advice would be to bring your toddler into contact with more people from an early age, be it family members or friends and suggest that they get involved in understanding and dealing with the child's needs.

Steven's second trip abroad

Steven was 15 months old at this time. He spent a month in Sri Lanka and a month in England. During this trip Steven had his MMR vaccination. He was still sociable and imitating people. He was still very active to the extent that I had to try four different types of harnesses and one wrist strap in an effort to keep him under control. He did not want to sit in a stroller, he did not want to be carried and he did not want to walk holding hands. The harness saw him trying to fly, the wrist strap was easily taken off, and he managed very easily to wriggle out of the straps in the stroller.

This trip marked a major change in Steven. On our return, the question asked by a number of friends was, *"why is he ignoring me?"* This was the beginning, where Steven gradually started to isolate himself, pull himself away from people and rejected any sort of interaction or affection. However, he was a happy child. At the onset of his oddness, he changed from a hyperactive child, who was happy in the company of people, to a child who was constantly looking to isolate himself from other children and adults.

Although Steven tried to reject affection, I insisted on hugs from him and did not let him get away from me until I had had a nice hug from him. Furthermore, this was the point when he seemed to lose interest in his toys.

Moving house
We moved from an apartment into a large house with a garden when Steven was two years old. This was in an area known as Mirdiff, a few miles from the centre of Dubai. At the time, this felt like it was the right decision for Steven but, unfortunately, it was not. The ample space meant that Steven was able to wander off anywhere to be on his own. He isolated himself

completely. The resistance to people and disinterest in his toys became very, very noticeable. He simply lost interest in his toys and people altogether.

The one and only interest that was retained was in watching Disney videos. He became more difficult to manage as his lack of understanding was becoming more apparent. Consequently I looked at local nurseries and managed to find one that was happy to take Steven on as long as I stayed with him. I observed Steven again, very closely, and compared him with other children who had speech delay. This was the time when my concerns meant that I had to know for sure if he had any problem that was causing the speech delay. I didn't expect it to be anything too serious or thought that whatever it was it could be fixed. Shortly after, an appointment was made to have Steven assessed by a developmental paediatrician.

Is it or isn't it Autism?
We arrived at the clinic where Steven was to be assessed. We sat in the waiting area ready to see the paediatrician who was an hour late. This gave me time to read through leaflets that were in the area outlining various conditions associated with child development. Amongst other topics I found a leaflet on Autism. I read through the leaflet, which had me thinking. Somehow, while reassuring myself it couldn't be possible. I asked the receptionist if she had any more information on the subject and I was given a fairly thick file that had more information on Autism, which I scanned through while waiting for the paediatrician to arrive. I was beginning to feel extremely concerned for

my son. My thoughts at this point were:

> *"Is my child Autistic?"*
> *"Could he be Autistic?"*
> *"No he couldn't be."*

The paediatrician finally arrived and Steven had a ½ hour assessment. She watched Steven play and asked me various questions regarding Steven's behaviour and development to date. She mentioned the word Autism to me but said that she couldn't be sure until Steven had a hearing test.

I must admit that I was very angry and observed that Autism should not be mentioned in circumstances such as this until such time that she was certain of a diagnosis. Looking back, I note that this particular paediatrician was extremely unprofessional in her approach as she showed a total lack of understanding in dealing with the situation. Most professionals in the medical field would not mention the word Autism, until they had all the facts together and were absolutely certain of the diagnosis.

Following the session, I left the clinic and drove back with Steven, feeling completely empty and with so much pain while thinking and feeling that my child cannot be Autistic. This was the first time that I had been truly enlightened to the condition and what it meant for the parent and the child. Although, having watched the movie "Rain Man", in which, Dustin Hoffman played the role of an Autistic adult, I did not want to accept it for my child. I was alarmed, where I felt a great deal of sadness during the movie. What created the strongest impression on my mind was that the Autistic adult Raymond Babbit could not fit into society and had to return to the institution, where he was drugged and kept happy. I thought to myself, I never want this for Steven. I had a 45-minute traumatic drive home with my adorable son sat in his seat at the rear completely oblivious to anything that was going on.

Autism hadn't been confirmed and friends and family did not want to accept it. I went into bookshops to read up on Autism. I found that the book shops in Dubai had very little reading material on the subject of Autism. When I did find any information it was generally a brief outline on Autism in a book on child development. I didn't want people to notice what I was reading as I felt ashamed, embarrassed and upset, that I moved away from people to ensure that no-one noticed what I was reading. The word Autism felt like a bad word and I felt ashamed of it. I did not even dare ask for any assistance.

Following the initial assessment with the paediatrician, it was arranged for Steven to have a hearing test. This again was rather a task, as getting Steven off to sleep wasn't so easy. In an attempt to get Steven to sleep, the ENT (Ear Nose and Throat) specialist gave him a dose of Phenergen, which showed no effect. Eventually, he gave him four times the usual dose of Phenergen, which still did not have any effect on him. I have read and noticed over time, that Autistic children had adverse reactions to drugs and sedatives although; convincing medical people of this is so difficult. Steven finally fell asleep but only after being taken for a drive during his usual sleep time.

The hearing test was performed. Once Steven woke up he was more difficult and aggressive than he had ever been. I wondered what the Phenergen might have done to his system to cause such a negative reaction and felt awful that I hadn't had more control over refusing to let him have the drug. The results of the tests were ready a week later and I went back to see the same paediatrician with this report and other information regarding Steven, which I thought would be useful in the assessment.

The paediatrician looked at the results of the hearing test and seemed confused. I asked again "Is he Autistic?" Her response was I have to do a series of assessments to be certain and this will cost Dhs.6,500/- (approximately £1,000). Following such a casual response, I expressed my anger in letting her know that she put me through two weeks of trauma, together with sleepless nights and questioned her on why she didn't have an answer for me. I asked her the reason for mentioning the word Autism if she wasn't sure? Her reply was, "I should not have said it. He could be Autistic; he could have ADHD (Attention Deficit and Hyperactivity Disorder)."

At the end of the second visit, I asked the paediatrician if she had anything positive to say about my son to which she replied "Yes, the fact that he likes little things." I asked her what it meant and was told, "Time is up. Let us discuss it next time." I did not go back to this particular paediatrician!

I was extremely concerned for the future of my child which led me to return to the bookshops to find books on ADHD with less unease than when I was looking for information on Autism. Having read up on ADHD, I felt it wasn't as bad as Autism and hoped that he had this condition rather than Autism.

We had planned to travel to Australia and New Zealand over Christmas and arranged to have Steven assessed during this trip.

Confirmation of Autism

We stopped in Australia on our way to New Zealand. It was only when we arrived in Australia that I learnt that Steven's cousin, who was 13 years old, had already been diagnosed with ADHD. Steven's cousin, apart from being hyperactive, was functioning normally in every other way and was performing well in school. After learning this, the concerns were starting to grow. As a result, I began to watch Steven very closely, to observe his behaviour and understand him.

From Australia, we travelled to New Zealand where Steven was assessed by a developmental paediatrician in Auckland. He tested Steven as well as watched him play. Autism was confirmed. Steven was 2½ years old at the time, and since he was able to complete age appropriate puzzles, he was diagnosed as mildly Autistic. The paediatrician informed us that he would make himself available at the end of the day to speak to us regarding any concerns. However, once we met, his final comments were, *'don't expect much'*. At this point I refused to accept his words since I had never had to deal with a situation, where I couldn't find an answer to resolve a problem. Furthermore, during this trip I was to learn that Steven's grand dad and his great grand dad had both suffered from epilepsy. They had both led normal lives and Steven's great grand dad had shown an exceptional talent in music. I learnt that ADHD and epilepsy were both minor brain dysfunctions while Autism was a major brain dysfunction.

Following the visit the paediatrician arranged for Steven to have a test for Fragile X Syndrome, which would rule out any other concerns in addition to Autism. Taking Steven for this test was not only traumatic but needed four adults to hold down a determined 2½ year old. The test proved negative but Steven's diagnosis of Autism, mild or not, made me feel that my worst nightmare had come true.

Once Steven's diagnosis of Autism had been confirmed, we were put in touch with a speech therapist as well as "The Auckland Autistic Society." We met with the President of the Auckland Autistic society, who was a mother of a ten-year-old Autistic child. She briefed us on the subject and gave us general views on Autism. I was extremely depressed having learnt all this new information, which I could not accept as I was convinced that my child was only mildly affected and could not be so bad. At the end of our meeting when the mother of the Autistic child tried to hug me, I pulled away from her, as I wasn't ready to accept the Autism and the huge challenges that I was expected to face.

During this time, I was greatly in need of mental and emotional support. This support was not available. We informed members of the family. I was even more hurt to learn that, to some members of the family, it was more important that I kept quiet about the Autism than that they should support me at a time of desperate need.

My love for Steven didn't change the way I felt about him. Rather, it made me more determined to do everything that I possibly could for him. Steven needed me and I him. We did everything together. We had very rarely been separated from each other and I was ready to give it my best shot.

Return to Dubai after the diagnosis

Steven was 2½ years old at this time and my priorities were to arrange Speech & Language Therapy as well as to find a suitable nursery setting. I began taking Steven to Speech Therapy for two, one hour, sessions a week, as well as to a playgroup twice a week. I informed the nursery, which Steven attended with myself as his helper, of the diagnosis, as we continued to attend the nursery. Shortly after, Steven's class teacher was due to go away for a month's holiday, at which time the head teacher asked if I could take the class for her. I advised her of the difficulty as Steven needed my one-to-one support. She let me know that they were "doing me a favour" in keeping Steven. I decided at this point to give it a go for Steven's sake. However, managing a class full of 2½ year olds together with Steven was hard. I tried it for a day but ended up with a severe migraine. I had to inform the head teacher that I couldn't do the job and removed Steven from such a negative environment. The move to Mirdiff, into a large spacious house, with a garden, now seemed the worst possible decision for Steven. There was a shortage of English nurseries in the area. I set up a work area in the house where I could teach Steven.

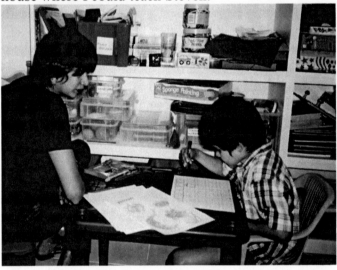

Teaching Steven at home

The idea of teaching Steven, which I took upon as a challenge was exciting. However, I only learnt the difficulties involved when I had to do it myself. I decided that Steven needed 100% motivation and an equal level of commitment from me. It was more than a challenge at first which meant that it was absolutely necessary that Steven felt secure and confident in my approach to teaching him. I recognised that building my child's confidence and trust was the key to helping him move forward. Steven was content, when there were no demands placed on him and when he was given everything that he wanted. Placing demands on him and imposing restrictions on his wants, turned into a battle of wills. I recognised that gaining any sort of compliance through a soft approach would not work for Steven, which led me to combine the soft and the hard approaches. I used the hard approach of the Lovaas method combined with Play Therapy, PECS (Picture Exchange Communication System) and Occupational Therapy to develop skills. The combination of a variety of methods seemed to be effective with Steven.

To teach Steven to sit on a chair to learn meant that he would scream for an hour. To get Steven to sit at the meal table with others resulted in a screaming session. As a result, I realised the significance of teaching Steven to sit as well as accept others. I learnt that what took place naturally in most children had to be taught to Steven and taught despite resistance. The combination of the different methods of teaching not only taught Steven skills involved in that particular activity, but helped him focus on life and his environment.

We worked on
* Sitting
* Developing eye contact
* Matching pictures
* Simple inset puzzles
* Threading reels
* Painting

Steven began to progress very slowly and although

progress was slow, I felt a great sense of satisfaction. I worked with Steven daily and he started to become a less tormented, happier child. At playgroup, whilst other mothers stood around chatting and drinking tea or coffee, I sat working with Steven. I helped with other children and found that other children joined Steven. All that mattered to me was to help Steven, see him learning and doing tasks that he could not have done before. Every little step was an achievement.

Once Steven learnt to sit, we worked on many activities. We used play activities to help develop awareness of himself and of others. I chose materials and objects that took his interest in order to motivate him, whilst making learning fun. I never felt that Steven had shut me out as I discovered numerous ways in which to enter his world. Steven enjoyed music, dance and animals. These were good starters as we spent a fair bit of time between activities, dancing to music and playing with toy animals. In addition, we worked on objects to help him learn to differentiate, and to learn that, different objects had different textures which he could feel.

Developing motivation in Autistic children
Autistic children's development does not correspond with what is expected of their age. Consequently, there is no measure to gauge the level of progress and what could be expected of the future. The level of expectation must not be pushed too far beyond the level of ability, which could result in the child being distressed, while reducing the level of motivation. Therefore, a comfortable and secure learning

environment, with dedicated teaching will help encourage learning, in relation to the child's level of ability. Offer support in enabling the child to progress at a comfortable pace within their capabilities.

Play and social development takes place during the early stages of an infant's life. They start with imitating others while building up to imaginative and symbolic play. They learn the meaning of interaction and recognition, which further develops into an awareness of themselves. They learn that things can be perceived differently by others and develop an understanding of the meaning of social acceptance. Encouraging learning through play will aid your Autistic child's development in accepting the world outside their own. Play can be taught well through symbolic play, where toys are used to represent real life activities. For example, using a toy train set to move the trains along the track. These activities help towards laying the foundation in understanding a more complex world.

Autistic children experience difficulties in engaging in play activities due to the complexities involved in the use of language, understanding the thoughts and feelings of others and in understanding imaginative play. As a result, they seek comfort in engaging in repetitive or obsessive play. An Autistic child will require guidance in learning to play in an appropriate manner using toys.

We were different
Steven's Autism meant that he was left out of all the play group children's birthday parties. At first it didn't matter. However, as time went on, it turned out to be a regular occurrence, where Steven was the only child left out. This made me feel stronger for Steven with the thought of not having time for anyone who didn't have time for us.

We had a few good friends who accepted Steven and loved him *"No matter what"* his condition meant. Their children too accepted Steven, allowing him the opportunity to feel comfortable and secure in being around other people. These friends were completely unselfish and ready to help at a time of need.

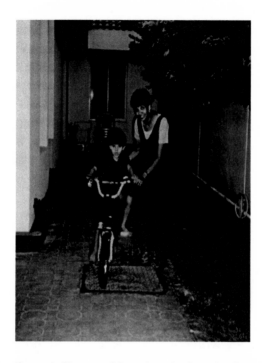

A lack of specialist teaching for Autism in Dubai
Dubai was lacking in what it had to offer towards teaching Steven. As a result, I taught myself through reading as well as through my observations of Steven. In addition, I used my own techniques that I found to be effective in teaching Steven.

Steven was nearly four years old, when I felt it necessary that he learnt to fit into a school environment. Mirdiff had nothing to offer, which meant it was time to move again. This time Steven's needs meant a small bungalow type of house, with a garden just big enough for Steven. During this time Steven had started to become comfortable with being around people. The new home did not give him much opportunity to be on his own. The garden ran right around the house, which meant that if he were to go outside he could still be seen from any room in the house. Similarly, he would know that he was being watched. The area was good for amenities with plenty of nursery schools within a five minutes drive from home. However, having checked on as many nurseries as possible, it became evident that no nursery was prepared to offer him a place.

I finally found a special needs centre in the area that was happy to offer him a place. Dubai does not publicise special needs schools or therapy centres which meant that finding such a place wasn't easy. Whilst Steven attended this centre in the mornings, I worked with him at home in the afternoons. Steven had spent most part of a year at this centre and while I was still working with him at home in the afternoons, it was clear that he hadn't learnt anything at the centre.

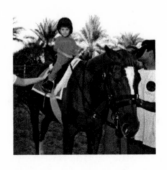

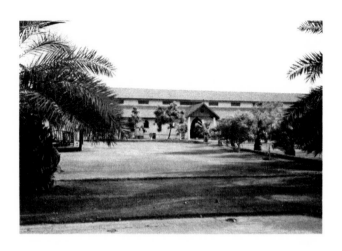

In addition, I took Steven horse riding and swimming as well as on regular visits to the park and a jungle gym. Horses being one of Steven's obsessions meant that he really looked forward to this activity, which he more than enjoyed. He had developed a natural stride through his riding lessons at the age of 4 years. The perfectly maintained RDAD (Riding for the Disabled Dubai) stables were located surrounded by lush green, which created a relaxed and calming environment together with an immense therapeutic appeal. Steven not only learnt to ride while developing an awareness of himself through balance and coordination, but further developed his language skills through commands that he learnt to give the horses. He enjoyed imitating the sounds made by the horses and was overjoyed to learn that the horses responded to him by repeating the sounds.

Concern over Educational provision in Dubai

While Steven was placed at a special needs centre in Dubai, I was rather concerned that he wasn't given the specialist attention that he desperately needed. Therefore, I decided that he needed a more up to date assessment. We arranged for Steven to be assessed by two reputable specialists in the UK, in August of 1998.

The updated assessment stated that Steven was severely Autistic with a severe receptive language disorder. Steven was 4½ years old at this time. The report which was written following the assessment was true and accurate. I was offered advice on managing behaviours, together with a list of books to assist me with home teaching. This was the first time that I had met anyone who was so clued up on the subject while being able to recognise Steven's individual needs. Following the assessment, I felt a sense of relief with the thought that there was light at the end of the tunnel. We returned to Dubai where Steven continued to attend the special needs centre in the mornings while working with myself in the afternoons.

Preparing for Riana's birth

Steven was nearly five years old when I was expecting my second child. I made best use of the time I had and did as much work as possible with Steven. We had plenty of fun and Steven was now a happy, more focused child. Furthermore, I had thought of ways to introduce the new baby to Steven. Steven was taught to stroke my tummy and say, "Steven's baby" which was taught throughout the pregnancy.

The amount of work which had to be done with Steven meant that I was left with very little time to prepare for the birth of my new baby. The question was asked if I was concerned about my second child being Autistic. My answer was, "if it is, I will be able to offer this baby a very good start in life, but I know it isn't." I felt positive energy right through the pregnancy and knew that this baby was going to be ok.

The date for the birth of the baby was nearing, which led me to prepare instructions for all concerned in dealing with Steven. The instructions were clearly written out step by step to avoid any confusion in communicating with or caring for Steven.

An incident in Dubai - Can grandmas cope?
Four days prior to the birth of Riana was when grandma from Sri Lanka arrived to help with the new baby. Grandma was asked to watch Steven in the garden one evening whilst I got dinner prepared. Shortly after I had started the preparations, I heard a scream from grandma. I ran outside to find that Steven had pulled a chair, unbolted the gate and run into the middle of the road. There was a pile of soil on an island that had taken Steven's interest. I asked grandma to run to Steven and bring him back, but she was in shock and could not act. So it was that while being nine months pregnant I was forced to run across a busy main road avoiding and stopping traffic to get to Steven. Fortunately, Steven was removing his sandals and getting ready to climb the pile of soil when I picked him up and brought him back home.

By this time, Steven's diagnosis was known. My advice would be to have the gates securely bolted to avoid any danger to the child and ensure that the person dealing with the child is experienced in predicting and dealing with the situation.

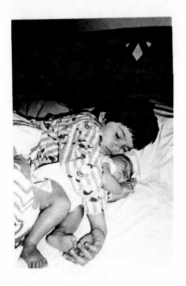

Impact of Riana's birth on Steven
Riana was born and Autism was not a concern. She was alert from day one. Until this time, I had very rarely been separated from Steven for long, which resulted in my starting to miss him. I must admit that following the joy of the new baby, what delighted me most was hearing the sounds of Steven walking along the corridor of the American Hospital to visit us. I knew that I was going to see him soon. Steven entered the room and he immediately approached me for a cuddle when he noticed his baby sister. He looked at her and seemed fascinated by her and her movements. He kept

attempting to touch her while pulling his hand away at each instant that she squirmed. From this time onwards his interest was Riana.

I returned home from hospital. Having been away for two days, I needed to get back on track with teaching Steven. However, on my return I was first rejected by Steven, following which he hugged me and sobbed while looking for comfort from me. This was a very normal reaction which I experienced for the first time in Steven.

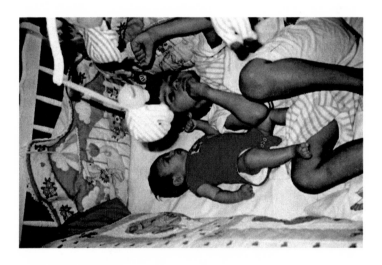

The following morning Steven got into Riana's cot and he continued to do so at every opportunity that came his way. He always made it a point to get in at the foot end of the cot where he sat watching his baby sister while being careful not to step on her. Steven now kept me on my toes as I was concerned that he could fall on the baby. Steven seemed to enjoy watching Riana at all times. He watched her in her car seat, in her carrycot, in her cot and her rocker chair. He attempted to carry her a few times, where he dumped her on the sofa or his bean bag, when she indicated distress through her cry of panic. I was only relieved that he didn't dump her on the hard tiled floor. Furthermore, he joined me in singing nursery rhymes to Riana while constantly asking for baby.

Riana took an interest in Steven from a very early age too. She was sat in her rocker chair at three days old watching Steven work, following his movements using her eyes before she had learnt to crawl or walk. She seemed to be fascinated by watching Steven on the trampoline while he too watched her while she lay in her play pen. Steven's level of activity meant that Riana's head was moving all the time while being alert to the possibility of being picked up by her brother.

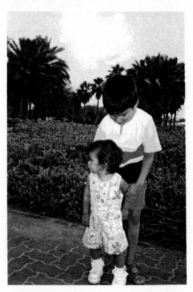

As time went on, the concerns regarding Steven's future kept growing. The staff at the special needs centre confessed that they were not geared to teaching Autistic children. Consequently, I withdrew Steven from the centre and started to educate him at home once again. During this time, I had Riana to attend to as well. In order to give both children sufficient time it was necessary to hire extra help. I worked with Steven for half a day throughout the week and hired help and trained them to work the rest of the day. In addition, I had help with Riana, which meant the day could run smoothly with regard to Steven's learning. Steven was doing very well while learning at home, which led me to believe that he had the potential to achieve a great deal more if, we were to return to the UK.

The facilities available towards teaching Autistic children in Dubai, as well as the place itself concerned me. Dubai was not the place for an Autistic child to learn. Life itself was artificial lacking, in many of the day-to-day activities in life, which most children learn from. People taking walks, or walking dogs or Mums pushing buggies were not often seen. I could not expect Steven to make sense of what was illustrated in the children's story books. Life in Dubai suited most other expatriates, but it did not suit me or Steven. The priority was to do what was needed for Steven, which meant taking a stand to return to the real world. My only disappointment in leaving Dubai was that Steven was going to miss out on his horse riding, which he enjoyed.

My life in Dubai, although it was never idle, was free of any of life's hardships. I recognised that returning to the UK meant managing the two children on my own without a fraction of the support that I was used to in Dubai. However, I was sure I could handle it. I had made my decision based on my faith in the system, which was going to provide Steven with a chance to achieve his full potential. Having recognised Steven's potential through his learning at home, I felt that given the opportunity anything was achievable.

I was clear that it was the correct decision and wrote to the Local Education Authority, in the area in which we were to return to, providing a detailed report on Steven and requesting a place at a suitable Autistic school. Shortly afterwards, we received a response from the LEA stating that a suitable place had been allocated to Steven.

Having experienced such expert advice at the time of Steven's assessment in the UK in 1998, I was certain it was the right decision. It was only after we had returned and settled that I learnt that this level of expertise is hard to come by and I acknowledged the reputation of the two specialists in the field of child development and psychology.

We returned to the UK in July 2000 with Steven and his baby sister Riana. Steven was stimulated by the environment, which had a great deal to offer in terms of understanding the world around him. Following our return, we visited the school in which Steven had been offered a place and received a tour of the school.

Steven seemed comfortable and eager to explore his surroundings. During our visit, one of the teachers suggested that Steven remained in the classroom with the other children until it was time for us to leave. Having been taught at home, using a strict and consistent approach, meant that Steven was able to fit into the classroom setting comfortably. At this time, I was not aware of the availability of alternative schools and hoped that this school would help Steven learn and show further progress.

Steven, Riana and I remained in the UK, while Dad returned to work in Dubai.

Concerns over educational provision in the UK
Steven started at the school for Autistic children where he appeared to have settled comfortably for the first term. However, the lack of input indicated that Steven wasn't making any progress. Although, a detailed report of Steven's achievements in Dubai had been sent to the school, prior to him starting at the school, they were not able to come close to reaching the level that he already had.

Shortly after Steven started at the school, he was assessed by the LEA's Educational Psychologist, the school's Speech and Language Therapist as well as his Class Teacher. The reports written by these specialists had drawn heavily from the original report that had been prepared by me in Dubai while any additional comment proved that Steven was functioning at a very basic level. It was clearly evident that Steven had not been assessed accurately. At this point, I felt it necessary to work closely with the school. The school ignored my input and saw it as interference, rather than a genuine interest in helping my child. The parent/teacher partnership, which is absolutely essential in the education of an Autistic child, was a mockery.

Steven was in a class of eight children, supervised by four adults. As time went on it was becoming even more apparent that Steven was not making any progress. Steven needed extra Speech & Language Therapy as well as a one-to-one support assistant to work with him throughout the day.

The LEA continuously refused my request for the extra provision that Steven so desperately needed. Their view was that Steven did not need the additional support and they continuously stated that the school shared this view. I felt frustrated with the knowledge of what Steven was capable of achieving and felt helpless as I had a toddler to take care of as well. Unlike in Dubai I did not have the extra home help. As a result, I allowed the school more time to show progress in Steven. *(The story continues in the chapter 3 with the battle for rights to education)*

CHAPTER FOUR

COMMITMENT TO EDUCATION

Choosing a suitable educational environment

Parents want what's best for their children and struggle to give them the best. Whether it is in a mainstream environment, special needs school, or a home based programme the decision should be based on what is most suited to meet your child's individual needs. The choice should be made based on the child's ability, which should be determined according to the age and level of development. Needs may vary depending on mobility, co-ordination, language development and the ability to cope in a chosen environment.

Every Autistic child is an individual. Therefore, it is absolutely essential that their individual needs are met. Learn the value of unfolding your child's true potential by addressing the individual needs, once a diagnosis has been made. In addition learn to understand your child and his/her needs, when choosing a suitable educational environment. This means that your child should not be positioned in an educational establishment that cannot cater to his/her needs, rather that the educational environment is tailored to fit the individual educational needs of the child.

An effective curriculum for an Autistic child is one that is developed to address their specific cognitive needs. Seeing the world as they do and working on areas of specific difficulty to help them learn and progress within their capabilities.

Effective strategies for teaching children with cognitive and communication disorders

- Ensure the child is attending to the instructions before you start speaking - Observe the child's eyes and move close to face the child and stay in line with the child's eye level.
- Give clear auditory and visual information - Avoid any abstract or confusing information. Speech should be very clear allowing the child to process what has been said at his/her level of functioning.
- Remove any distractions that may cause inattention or inability to focus from the working environment.
- Teach at the child's level of learning ensuring the steps are broken into achievable tasks.
- Repetition will be required to give the child an opportunity to pick up and process what has been taught aurally or visually. The child will need to be tested to understand the child's level of attention and the amount of information that has been absorbed.
- In the likelihood that the child has difficulty making sense of what has been said, it will be necessary to encourage learning by using a prompt until the message is clearly understood and the child is able to respond independently.
- The environment should be clear of any background sounds that could be seen as likely to distract the child.
- Support and encourage attempts to communicate by responding quickly and consistently.
- Constantly reinforce what has been learnt while moving on to the next stage. Mix topics that interest the child between areas that take more motivation.

This will help reduce boredom as well as help the child stay on task for longer periods of time.
- Encourage the child to participate in a group situation - Help the child learn to pay attention to other children as well as learn the rules of turn taking.
- Minimise frustration and create motivation by simplifying steps to suit the child's level of learning.

TYPES OF EDUCATIONAL PROVISION

- Mainstream school with a one-to-one classroom support.
- Autistic unit attached to a mainstream school.
- Mainstream school without one-to one support.
- Autistic school catering specifically for Autistic children.
- Language unit catering for children with language and communication difficulties.
- Home based education.

A school is responsible for preparing the 'IEP' (Individual Educational Plan), which outlines a list of skills the child is expected to learn. Once drafted it is discussed and agreed between the school and the parents and targets are set accordingly. The main focus of this programme is to develop skills that are required for the child's future development.

In addition to these choices of education, Autistic children depending on their specific needs may need

Speech & Language Therapy, Occupational Therapy and Physiotherapy.

When teaching Autistic children a great deal of emphasis needs to be placed on the strengths and interests of the child. Motivate and further encourage their learning, though creating strategies to support that strength. To be certain of the child's learning style, a series of tests using different methods can be used. Tests can be carried out through the use of books, pictures, puzzles, toys, drawings, computers, music and dance. Once the child's learning style has been identified the child can be taught using the most suited method of learning. Skills learnt on a one to one basis will need to be generalised across the board, through social and everyday activities.

Mainstreaming an Autistic child means fitting into a regular educational setting without the additional support of a specially trained teacher. This approach works well for a child who is ready and able to fit into the setting where they learn more appropriate skills from better role models, as well as receive more opportunities for social interaction. However, in mainstreaming, the child has to have the abilities and the strengths expected, as a child of the same age, or the potential to reach that level. A child who is not ready to be mainstreamed could result in an outcome which could be harmful to the Autistic child as well as the rest of the class. A point to bear in mind is where disruptive behaviour stems from and that is through confusion or an inability to cope. Therefore, the prime focus should be to place an Autistic child in a setting that suits their needs taking into consideration their educational requirements, together with their level of physical and emotional development. The environment should be altered if necessary to achieve those needs.

METHODS USED IN TEACHING AUTISTIC CHILDREN

- *LOVAAS*
- *ABA*
- *PECS*
- *TEACCH*
- *Speech Therapy*
- *Sign Language / Makaton*
- *Occupational Therapy*
- *Sensory Integration Therapy*
- *Play Therapy*
- *Holding Therapy*
- *Dolphin Therapy*
- *Option Therapy*
- *Facilitated Communication*
- *Physical Therapy*
- *Computer Software*
- *Vision Training*
- *Irlene Lenses*
- *Relationship Development Intervention*
- *Social Skills Training*

Other treatments
- *Mega Vitamin Therapy*
- *Folic acid*
- *Vitamin B6*
- *Fish oil*
- *Gluten - Casein free diet*
- *Dymethyglycin supplements (DMG)*
- *Secretin injection*
- *Cranial Osteopathy*
- *Singing*
- *Vestibular Stimulation*

The LOVAAS method
A method developed by professor Ivor Lovaas at UCLA to treat Autistic children. It is a behaviour modification programme which uses positive reinforcements to reward appropriate behaviours. This is achieved through praise or a favourite activity, while in contrast negative behaviours are eliminated through penalising the action, for example by removing the reward or time out. The programme places an emphasis on developing attention, gaining social skills, understanding concept formation, developing language skills, meaningful play and life skills. The ME book which was written by professor Lovaas in 1981 describes the method. Behaviours which interfere or detract from learning are discouraged and eliminated through this approach.

ABA (Applied Behaviour Analysis)
A highly intensive method of teaching which focuses on behaviour and skills. It is a behaviour modification

programme using rewards to motivate by rewarding appropriate behaviour to encourage further learning. The programme is highly structured and intensive, delivered on a one to one basis. Skills are broken down to the simplest steps in order to assist the child to learn. Tasks are achieved one step at a time before they are mastered. The programme focuses on achieving skills through repetition, reinforcement, shaping, prompting, fading and extinction. As the Autistic child's learning is complex the priorities are given to all areas of learning which include language skills, social skills, play skills, physical skills, gross and fine motor skills as well as life skills. The prompts and reinforcements will be gradually reduced until the child is able to learn without rewards. A major part of the learning of our environment is absorbed through our senses while auditory learning is an essential part of that learning. Language skills are seen as critical for independent functioning. Therefore, a well designed programme will help the child learn through teaching the child to transfer the learnt skill to different situations.

PECS (Picture Exchange Communication System)
A system developed to assist non-verbal individuals with Autism to initiate their needs by exchanging a picture for the item that they desire. This is done where the child gives a picture of what they want to an adults hand after which, the adult exchanges it for the desired item. Symbols and words are also used to express feelings and needs.

TEACCH (Treatment and Education of Autistic and Related CommuniCation Handicapped children)
A method developed to help structure the day of an Autistic child through the use of pictures and photographs or words. A process that allows the transition from one activity to another to flow smoothly. It minimises the confusion of what takes place next by using a schedule to explain the day. The child will be given a task to complete. For example, matching pictures and once the task is complete the picture of the task will be placed in a box. Laminated pictures, symbols and words are also used to respond to a question or to request something the child desires. The TEACCH method works mainly on the child's terms. It would benefit Autistic children to a greater extent if the method is used in conjunction with a behaviour modification programme.

SPEECH & LANGUAGE

Speech Therapy
Teaching language to an Autistic child is more than just teaching speech. It involves teaching language to be used in a meaningful way to communicate effectively in various situations. Speech & Language Therapy is used to assist a child with Autism to develop language and communication skills. The therapy is delivered depending on the level and ability to communicate. Oral exercises are used to stimulate language development while objects, pictures and real life situations are used to develop comprehension of language.

Typical speech and language development
The first three years of a child's development are the most intensive period of speech and language development. Skills are learnt and absorbed best in a world filled with stimulation from the senses as well as exposure to social and everyday situations. The emergence of speech and language is driven by a desire to communicate and interact with the world.

The first signs of communication appear when an infant cries to express hunger, tiredness, a need to be held or comforted or to express a sign of discomfort. Newborns learn to recognise the sound of their mother's voice and seek comfort from knowing that she is there. Research suggests that most babies recognise the sound of their native language by the age of six months.

An infant will start with "cooing" moving onto babbling followed by jargon (which sounds like real words but are words that are made up) to saying a few words with meaning. As language develops they start linking words together and learn that words represent objects, feelings, thoughts and actions. From three years to five years of age they will master the rules of language. Phonology being sounds used in speech, morphology being the formation of words, syntax being sentence formation, semantics being meaning of word and sentence, prosody being intonation and rhythm of speech and pragmatics being effective use of language.

Speech & Language problems in Autism
The cause for communication problems in Autism is not known, but experts believe that it is due to a variety

of conditions that takes place either before, during or after birth which impacts on mental development.

A child who has learnt the meaning of language will use language to communicate the message they are sending which will be easily interpreted by the listener. They express themselves through language which leaves no room for confusion or frustration on the part of the speaker or the listener. The activity becomes two way where the message is sent to the listener who receives and processes the message and sends a response using language. In this process the universal language helps reason, negotiate, comply or even argue. The inability to communicate through language or gesture presents an obstacle to the messenger as well as the receiver. The messenger ends up feeling frustrated and confused which leads to communicating through bizarre or aggressive behaviour. To help a child with severe communication difficulties requires a good interpreter who has the ability to train themselves to observe and comprehend non verbal communication associated with behaviour and mood.

Encouraging speech development
Language is the most crucial skill in child development. Once language emerges, many of the other areas of development fall into place. Without the support of language, helping a child link the pieces of the world together in a pictorial sense is almost impossible. Language helps in recalling what has been seen, while enabling us to make sense of that vision.

Parents are most concerned if their child will ever

develop speech. With appropriate intervention, children with Autism can learn to use language to some extent. As communication is a crucial part of living in our world, it is vital to place an emphasis in encouraging speech development from an early age. Methods of use that have shown to be effective are:

- *Sign language*
- *Picture exchange communication system (PECS)*
- *Applied behaviour analysis (ABA)*
- *Singing*
- *Vestibular stimulation*

Sign language

A system of communication using the movement of hands which is easier than using speech for children with severe auditory and language disorders. Parents could learn to sign when talking to their child. It is referred to as 'simultaneous communication' or 'signed speech' which, will encourage and increase the chances of spoken language.

OCCUPATIONAL THERAPY

A therapy used to help Autistic children perform tasks which are required for gaining life skills. It could involve learning activities through play such as self care and dressing up. An Occupational Therapist will implement a program to assist your child in developing strengths and interests to build developmental skills.

Developing attention span

A child who continuously fidgets while not paying

attention to what he/she is doing will not be able to learn effectively. An OT will look at what motivates your child to sit still and will help the child keep calm and ready to learn.

Developing Sensory processing skills
A child needs to pick up information from all the senses and use them in an effective manner. The senses together with body movement and awareness are registered by sensory receptors, processed in the brain and acted upon in a way that the child functions in the most efficient way.

Fine and Gross motor skills
Many children with Autism display difficulty in learning skills such as drawing, using scissors, buttoning clothes or stringing beads. Autistic children will need help in developing the strength of the small muscles in their hands in order to help with the dexterity and co-ordination which are required for developing many life skills. Working on gross motor skills helps develop strength and awareness of the larger muscles: these skills could involve throwing and catching a ball, hopping, kicking a ball, jumping and climbing.

Activities involving daily living
Children are confronted with many daily living tasks which include eating, using utensils, drinking from a cup, dressing and undressing, washing hands, having a bath or shower, using the toilet and general personal hygiene.

Visual perceptual skills

A skill which teaches a child to learn the ability to perceive differences and relationships between objects. This includes learning to build blocks, do puzzles and understand geometry. The aim is to help the child to understand and fit into the world around them. A skill that is a must in helping a child feel physically and emotionally secure.

Sensory Integration Therapy

A treatment which assists a person with Autism to improve the way in which their nervous system receives sensory input. It is usually carried out by an Occupational Therapist. Autistic children require this method of therapy as they could be over sensitive to touch, sound and light, be hyper active, clumsy with movements, unable to control self or calm self and show signs of speech delay. The typically developing brain integrates the sensors automatically. The Autistic brain requires a great deal of input in achieving the integration of the sensors, where the accuracy cannot be guaranteed. The process which is distorted results in learning and development being delayed. Sensory integration helps a child by training all the sensors to coordinate and work together. Each of our sensors teaches us different information about ourselves and the world. It is often confusing or difficult for an Autistic child to process all the information at the same time. The coordination of the sensors are balanced in a way to help the Autistic child process information about who they are, the world around them and what takes place in that world.

Who would benefit from sensory integration therapy?

- A child who has difficulty gripping and using a pencil
- A child who has difficulty engaging in appropriate play using toys
- Has difficulty with coordination to dress one's self and general self care tasks
- Has difficulty coping with movement making everyday fun and playground activities a fear
- Hyperactive or over active children who are seen as a danger to themselves
- Tactile defensive children

Tactile defensiveness

An Autistic individual who is tactile defensive indicates over sensitivity to touch or is distressed through contact with everyday situations. This creates a further barrier towards learning as individuals associated with such symptoms resist using their hands effectively. They avoid contact with textures and touch certain textures with just their finger tips. The avoidance of textures blocks out acceptance of sensory stimulation. Typically this is demonstrated by:

- A child who dislikes being touched or hugged
- A child who dislikes textures, seams or labels on clothes
- A child who dislikes getting dirty or dislikes contact with sand or grass on bare skin

For example, Steven first indicated resistance to physical contact by pulling himself away during his baby years. However, he soon learnt to enjoy the sensation of touch, through daily massage which he received throughout his baby and toddler years. He also resisted any form of restraint. The first hurdles were when he rejected the straps on his high chair, his stroller, the car seat belt and the seat belt on a flight. Each situation resulted in a battle where he refused to comply. However, with the road and air travel requirements for seat belts which are clearly necessary for Steven's safety, I felt that the battle was necessary and he had to comply. Once he learnt to associate the action starting with the belt a bit loose and gradually tightening it as time went on, he learnt to ask to have his belt on and he has now learnt to fasten it himself. In addition Steven found wearing a belt with his trousers extremely distressing. He would get aggressive when made to wear one. He would remove it continuously and choose to go out with his trousers falling down. The conflict went on for a while until one day he got aggressive and out of control and hurt me. On that occasion, I dealt with the behaviour by insisting on staying in while ignoring him. He asked to go out using any language or method of communication he could find, to let me know that he wanted to go out. I ignored him for most part of the day and by the end of the day he brought me his belt and said 'belt on please'. He started wearing the belt loose and gradually tightening it allowed him time to accept it himself. He has now fully accepted and is comfortable with it.

Play Therapy
Activities are based on play to encourage the child to learn as well as assess their ability in all cognitive

related areas. Toys and methods of play are used at home to encourage interaction and assist development in children who cannot learn in a normal way.

Holding Therapy
A form of therapy where the child is continuously held or hugged in order to teach them to accept the feeling of touch as well as a means of encouraging eye contact.

Dolphin Therapy
A swim with the dolphins has been reported to have a dramatic effect on the behaviour and development of Autistic children. Close contact with dolphins is said to stimulate the brain and boost a child's ability to learn. Scientists have discovered that when a dolphin comes into close contact with a human that there is greater harmony between the left and right sides of the brain, which is said to be caused by the dolphin's sonar.

Option Therapy
A home based programme involving the parents to teach through play. The programme follows the child's own behaviours and motivators in order to get through to the child's world.

Facilitated Communication
A technique that involves the adult/facilitator offering physical support to the child using hand over hand guidance. The child uses the facilitators hand as a guide to move his/her hand to request a desired object or activity.

Physical Therapy
Children with Autism who show a lack of understanding of body awareness can be helped through Physical Therapy.

Computer Training
Computer software specifically designed to help children with developmental disabilities have been effective in helping Autistic children. www.llsys.com

Vision Training
Many Autistic individuals have difficulty focusing on themselves as well as the environment. The problems are due to a limited attention span showing easy distractibility, using excessive eye movements, difficulty scanning or tracking movements, inability to catch a ball, stumbling over when climbing stairs or walking on tip toes. A programme which involves wearing prism lenses and performing visual motor exercises is said to reduce or eliminate many of the problems associated with vision.

Irlene Lenses
Coloured tinted lenses. An individual who is hypersensitive to particular types of lighting which could include fluorescent lighting, bright sunlight, certain colours or colour contrasts or have difficulty reading printed text, would benefit from wearing these lenses. The lenses are said to reduce the sensitivity as well as help improve reading skills.

Relationship Development Intervention
A method used to help children develop relationships with their parents, family and peers. The lack of social development being a core issue for most families with an Autistic child means that a great emphasis needs to be placed in this area of development. www.connectionscenter.com

Social Skills Training
An approach which involves teaching a child the skills required to cope with social situations. This involves developing and using appropriate eye contact, appropriate use of gestures, understanding the acceptable distance to stand at when talking to others and learning the meaning of non-verbal language. For example, body language, actions, gestures and expressions. Social skills are taught in different situations to allow the child to understand flexibility and adaptability in language and behaviour.

OTHER TREATMENTS

When deciding on a treatment it is vital to learn if a treatment has been proven effective and the extent of its effectiveness. A treatment that is not proving effective for your child is best stopped after the trial period, especially if it costs a great deal and involves a great deal of effort. It is recommended that only one treatment is tried at one time in order to gauge which one is proved to be effective or not.

Mega Vitamin Therapy
High doses of magnesium and vitamin B6 are said to

help reduce hyperactivity and behaviour problems. Steven received Super Nu-Thera Powder which contained high doses of the Magnesium and B6. The powder which was ordered from Kirkman Sales Company in the US was given to Steven for a period of two years with the hope that it would help develop his attention and further encourage his learning. It was administered in the required dose according to his weight by mixing it into yoghurt where he didn't mind the difference in taste. Although, at the time when we lived in Dubai, Steven indicated bouts of hyperactivity he was generally calm at other times. During this time Steven was enjoying his learning and while I cannot say if the treatment had any effect Steven continued to progress even after the treatment had been stopped.

Folic acid
Folic acid is said to help Autistic children as a symptom of deficiency in folic acid can cause hyperactivity. DMG (Dimethyglycine) causes an increased use of folic acid in the body resulting in a deficiency in folic acid. Dr.Bernard Rimland of the Autism Research Institute has recommended giving folic acid in conjunction with DMG. I gave folic acid to Steven together with DMG and Megavitamin therapy but recognised no obvious difference in him. The reason for introducing folic acid to Steven was an attempt to help with his inability to sleep at night.

Vitamin B6
A vitamin which is required for the production of serotonin as it affects mood, behaviours and sleep patterns.

Fish Oil - EyeQ

There have only been a few studies on the effectiveness of fish oil in the treatment of Autism. Some children who received the supplement had shown improvement in their overall health which included an improved sleep pattern, social interaction, reduced anxiety and improved eye contact. Furthermore, some scientists have stated that Autism, dyslexia, ADHD and Dyspraxia are a group of neurodevelopmental disorders which result from problems lying in the metabolism of EFAs. (Essential Fatty Acids) Their suggestion is further explained by the theory that individuals with Autism and related disorders have difficulty in converting Essential Fatty Acids from food to forms that are required for biochemical reactions. In addition it has been noted that omega-3 fatty acids seemed lower in individuals with Autism than in others.

Having tried the EyeQ form of fish oil supplement on Steven, I cannot say if it benefited him. I tried it on and off over a period of three months, but was concerned about Steven's reaction to it as he suffered a great deal of motion sickness at the time. However, I would recommend it as a health food supplement as I believe it cannot do the child any harm. The capsule form would be difficult for children who are unable to swallow. Therefore, the liquid form which is available in different flavours is easier to administer either by mixing it into juice or on its own.

Gluten - Casein free diet

Gluten is a protein found in wheat, barley and rye. Casein is a protein found in cows milk. It has been stated that in some cases the difficulty in breaking down these substances in the body could result in Autistic symptoms. I tried the two diets at different times. I first introduced Steven to the Casein free diet, which involved an intake of Soya milk instead of his regular milk. I gave him Soya milk which contained the RDA required daily dose of calcium for a period of six months, which didn't show any change in his Autism. He was enjoying his learning at the time and stopping the Soya milk made no difference. Although it was easy to introduce Steven to Soya milk, I wasn't keen on depriving him of his yoghurt and cheese which he really enjoyed. I tried the Gluten free diet for three months, but again, Steven showed no change once the diet was stopped. During this time in Dubai, the Gluten free section at the supermarkets had a limited range of products which made it difficult to continue. However, I found it almost impossible to do the two diets together.

Dimethyglycine supplements (DMG)
A food supplement with no known side effects. Parents have reported improvement in speech, eating habits, and behaviour patterns. It is found in small quantities in foods such as liver and brown rice. The reason for it not being classified as a vitamin is that there have been no specific deficiencies associated with a lack of it. Following Steven's diagnosis of Autism I ordered the 125mg DMG capsules from Kirkman Sales Company which required pulling apart and mixing with yoghurt as it was the most effective way of getting it into Steven. Steven was given the supplement for a two year period. While he was performing well with his learning

at the time it didn't indicate a change in his level of learning or behaviour once I stopped the DMG. Autism Research Institute has stated that DMG is responsible for enhancing the effectiveness of the immune system.

Secretin Injection

A hormone which is injected to test the bicarbonate levels in the blood in order to assess the function of the pancreas. The production of bicarbonate is required to neutralise the acids in the stomach. Other enzymes are also produced by the pancreas and stimulated by Secretin. It is used as a treatment for Autism due to the fact that enzyme production will break down harmful peptides that have been thought responsible for the cause of Autism. Secretin is manufactured and distributed by Fering laboratories in the USA It is difficult to obtain and very costly. We were living in Dubai when Secretin was brought to light, in 1999, as a treatment for Autism. Steven was four years of age. We were able to order it through the American hospital in Dubai. Steven was given four doses of Secretin at six week intervals made available to him by friends of the family who paid for the treatment. Steven was rather distressed, when he began to recognise the doctor who administered the Secretin. However, I hoped it would help Steven, but he showed no change except for a slightly improved sleep pattern.

Cranial Osteopathy

A treatment in which the skull bones are manipulated to treat head and spinal injury, mood disorders, cerebral palsy, hyperactivity, dizziness, dyslexia, and ear conditions.

Singing
Parents could encourage an interest in singing using a video or audio tape.

Vestibular Stimulation
Movement through swinging while Encouraging language.

Sandy Howarth

CHAPTER FIVE

EFFECTIVE SERVICES?

THE STATEMENTING PROCESS AND THE CODE OF PRACTICE

This chapter is to explain the ins and outs of the statementing process. A child who has difficulty learning according to what is expected of their age will be statemented. Steven was in a special needs school setting during the preparation of his Statement of Educational Needs.

Understanding the code of practice
The special educational needs code of practice has been drawn up to provide guidance to educational settings, State schools, LEAs and services. All parties responsible for recognising, identifying, and making the provision available for children with special educational needs, must and should follow to meet the needs of children. It clearly states that they must not ignore the guidance as set in the code.

The code of practice states that a child assessed with special educational needs has to be granted the provision. State schools and LEAs are required to recognise the code when dealing with children who have been assessed with special needs. The schools are required to work together with other services in supporting the LEA in providing the services.

The code of practice explains what special educational needs mean

The legal definition of 'Special Educational Needs' is when the child has disabilities with learning, which makes it hard for them to learn as compared with a child of the same age. A child with special educational needs may need additional support in learning to think, understand, develop physical skills, cope with sensory difficulties, cope with emotional and behavioural issues, and develop, language and social skills.

Suggests ways to deal with concerns over your child requiring special educational needs or not

In the likelihood that you are faced with concerns over your child's development, you should seek help straight away. Speak to a doctor or a health visitor who will be able to advice on the steps to take. If your child is in a school environment and you think your child may have special educational needs, but they have not yet been identified it is required that you speak to your child's class teacher and the SENCO (Special Educational Needs Co-ordinator). If your child is in a secondary school and you have concerns over your child requiring special needs you should speak to the child's class teacher the SENCO and the head teacher.

- Suggests ways to help your child
- Explains different educational settings and how they could help your child
- Explains the input of Educational Authorities and other services
- Explains your rights as a parent and the rights of the child - A process that many parents are faced with

is getting the provision that their child needs as opposed to the provision that the LEA decides is suitable. A parent has a right to choose which state school you wish your child to attend. This could be mainstream or a special education provision that your child is currently attending.

The LEA must agree with your preference as long as:

- The chosen school is suited for the child's age, ability, skills and special educational needs.
- Your child's presence will not disrupt the education of other children in that school
- Placing your child in the school is an efficient use of resources

If you wish your child to attend a special school which is not maintained by the LEA or an independent school that will be able to meet the child's needs, the LEA will have to consider your wishes before a decision is made. However, if there is a suitable state school, which is capable of meeting your child's needs, the LEA have no legal obligation to place your child at an independent school.

THE STATEMENT OF SPECIAL EDUCATIONAL NEEDS

The LEA will issue a Statement of Educational Needs in the event that a child's needs cannot be met within a regular school provision, where the additional support is required. This involves funds, specially trained staff, equipment and time.

A statutory assessment carried out by the Local Educational Authority (LEA). Parental involvement is a must as the LEA will often draft the SEN in a way that is unclear as well as confusing. The LEA will attempt to protect their funds by stipulating the minimal needs for the child. Parents must ask for the statement to be written clearly and accurately and ensure that provision is made specific before it is finalised.

There is a tendency amongst educational professionals to think that they know best and to try to patronise (at best) or refute (at worst), parental input. It is important to know that, under English law, parents have responsibility for their child's education and input is crucial.

The duration to issue a statement is 26 weeks
- 6 weeks - For a decision to be made with regard to a statement being required
- 10 weeks - To do the assessment and reach a decision on the statement
- 2 weeks - To outline the proposed statement
- 8 weeks - To finalise the statement

The first step is to evaluate your child's needs through assessments and find a school or educational environment, which is capable of meeting those needs. Visits to as many schools will give you a fair understanding of what is available and how they could meet your child's needs.

Autism is a complex mental condition with complex needs. Some schools may believe that they are capable of meeting your child's needs but as time goes on you may discover that this is not the case. Therefore, it is absolutely necessary that all available options are given careful consideration. During this time, parents may find it useful to look at ways of getting in touch with parents of other children within the chosen schools to learn of its effectiveness in dealing with "individual children" together with the school's capabilities in meeting those children's needs.

Furthermore, the available facilities within the school and the hours of allocation per child must be considered in gaining the suitable provision for your child. At times, when contacting other parents becomes difficult, it is best to speak to the National Autistic Society, who will be able to offer details with regard to getting in touch with other families and support groups. Ensure that the provision must meet the child's needs. For example, agreeing to fifteen minutes of Speech Therapy per week for a non verbal child will not help the child. Rather, it will further enhance the level of frustration within the child. It is not adequate.

The school, together with the parents, will request an assessment from the LEA for your child's educational needs. At this stage, The LEA is made aware of the child's special educational needs. Following the request, the LEA will write to the parents to suggest a formal assessment of the child's needs, together with a form, which parents are required to complete. This form asks parents for their views on the child's needs, behaviours, adaptability and social and communication needs.

Some parents, having just had a child diagnosed with

Autism, may still be in denial. They may unintentionally try to ease some of the emotional pain and stress of the long term responsibility, by not being completely honest with themselves of their child's needs. In such cases, the parents may paint a picture which indicates that their child's needs are not as intense as they are in reality. Obscuring the true picture serves to harm the child and acts in favour of the LEA, who will be more than pleased to offer the minimum support for your child. Therefore, in completing the form issued to the parents by the LEA, it is absolutely necessary to create a true and complete understanding of the child's educational needs, by giving examples of how the child deals with different situations. In order to support the parent's views, it is vital to gather any previous or early reports that may have been prepared by specialists following physical or psychological assessments. The parents are given twenty nine days to complete and return the form to the LEA.

A parent can ask for help from a named person, to be involved in the statementing process. This could be a friend or a professional who knows the child and the child's needs. The named person will be expected to be an active participant, to offer support as well as attend meetings.

In my experience, having not had a named person to support me throughout the statementing process, the LEA suggested and arranged an independent support worker. During my first meeting with the "independent" support worker, it was clearly evident that there was no sign of her acting in my son's best interest, rather a "front" which disagreed with my every view. However, her intentions were made obvious when her support was constantly in favour of the LEA's position. This rather disappointing start left an unpleasant feeling about the LEA, which made me determined to go through the process on my own.

Once the LEA receives the parents' views, together with additional reports, a decision will be made on whether or not to proceed with the assessment. The LEA will request reports from the child's current school, an educational psychologist, a medical report from the Health Authority, knowledge of the child and the child's needs from Social services, communication and language requirements from a Speech and Language Therapist, together with other educational requirements. To assist these professionals when making their observations of the child, the LEA will send copies of all information, provided by the parents, to all professionals involved, who will produce their own individual reports based on observations carried out at separate times. Once these reports have been completed, they will be sent to the LEA who will assess the information in each of the reports and decide if there is any special provision to be made.

Stages of Special Needs assessment
The Department for Education and Employments 1994 code of practice outlines the responsibilities of a school, if a child is recognised as having difficulty with learning or demonstrates behavioural issues that does not compare with other children of the same age.

The 5 stages of assessment

* **Stage one**

  The teachers, together with the head teacher, gather information regarding the child and identifies if the child has a special needs requirement. The parent assists in the identification of the needs. Information is gathered and the school consults with the (SENCO) (Special Educational Needs Co-ordinator).

* **Stage two**

  The SENCO who is responsible for any special needs provision draws up an Individual Education Plan (IEP). This is done through discussions with the child's parents and teachers. The IEP is a detailed plan, which outlines the targets that have been set for the child to achieve. This includes a date for a review to assess the level of progress that has been made.

* **Stage three**

  The SENCO brings in specialists who could advise for example, an Educational Psychologist or a specialist teacher. In the event the child is seen not to be making progress the SENCO or head teacher will discuss with the parent if they should instruct the Local Education Authority to do a statutory assessment. In addition they will look at the child's learning difficulties as well as their strengths to decide if different or extra educational support should be provided.

* **Stage four**

  Based on the information that has been put together about the child the LEA will look at the request for a statutory assessment. If the information provided is insufficient, they may request further information in order to assist them towards a decision.

- ***Stage five***
  The LEA considers whether to issue a statement of special educational needs and writes a statement of the help required and the targets to be met. The monitoring and the reviews are ongoing.

A parent has the right to ask for a statutory assessment at any stage. However, the LEA will look at evidence to show that they have taken into consideration the child's needs, at stage three, before a statutory assessment can go ahead.

A request for an assessment is considered by a panel made up of professionals with knowledge and experience of special educational needs.

Once a statement is issued, a copy will be sent to the parents outlining the child's educational needs, details of the sort of help that is required and how the help will be provided. Copies of all the supporting reports will be attached to the statement.

If the LEA decides not to issue a statement, they will write to the parents explaining why it wasn't issued. The parents have a right to appeal if they disagree.

What does the statement of educational needs contain
A statement of educational needs is expected to follow the format as set out by Government Regulations and is required to contain the information from part 1 through to part 6, that make up the statement of educational needs.

- ***Part 1***
Introduction of the child
The child's name, address and date of birth; The names and addresses of the child's parents; The child's language spoken at home and religion.

- ***Part 2***
Special educational needs (learning difficulties)
Details of the child's special educational needs as identified by the LEA during the statutory assessment, together with any reports received. These are attached as appendices to the statement.

- ***Part 3***
Special educational provision
The special educational provision that the LEA considers appropriate to meet the child's educational needs.
This should cover
- The objectives that the special educational provision should aim to meet
- The special educational provision that the LEA considers appropriate to meet the needs set in part 2 in order to meet the objectives
- The arrangements to be made for monitoring progress in meeting those objectives by setting

short term targets for the child's progress and reviewing the progress continuously

- **Part 4**

Placement

The type and name of school that the special educational provision set out in part 3 is to be made or the LEA's arrangements for the provision to be made otherwise than in school.

- **Part 5**

Non - Educational needs

Describes any non-educational needs that your child requires, as agreed between the LEA, the Health Services, Social Services and other agencies.

- **Part 6**

Non - Educational provision

Details of all relevant non-educational provision required to meet the non-educational needs of the child. The provision is agreed between the health service and/or social services and the LEA and includes the agreed arrangements for the provision.

The statement of educational needs is signed by the named officer. In addition, all advice obtained and taken into consideration during the assessment process, must be attached as appendices to the statement.

This must include
- Parental views
- Educational advice
- Medical report
- Educational psychologist's report

- Social services advice
- Other advice - Views of the child from other agencies whose advice is thought desirable.

Parents are given 15 days to respond to the statement. It is a must to comment on the proposals being made. Provide further evidence if necessary. The parents are expected to confirm that the draft statement includes the following:

All provision to be provided by the school or Authority or both
- The number of hours of help
- Any special therapy required
- Educational targets to be reviewed annually
- Any changes to the national curriculum
- A list of schools

The LEA will confirm the statement and send a copy to the parents, the head teacher and professionals involved in preparing the reports. If the parents are in disagreement with the statement they have the right to make a formal appeal. The information with regard to a formal appeal is sent to the parents with the statement.

Parental request for a statutory assessment
The LEA must comply with a parental request for a statutory assessment, unless they have made a statutory assessment within six months of the requested date or upon examining available evidence decide that a statutory assessment is not necessary. The LEA must take all parental requests seriously and take action immediately.

Assessments

It is necessary that annual assessments of your child are carried out throughout their school life. This would not only show if there has been any progress made but also show if the child's needs have changed in any way.

Who do you trust with assessments?

The accuracy of your child's assessment is an absolute must. Therefore, it is critical that you recognise your child's needs in order to enable you to gauge for yourself if the assessment is true and accurate. Alternatively you could pay to have independent reports done by reputed specialists.

BATTLE FOR RIGHTS TO EDUCATION

During the statementing process, which involved Steven's needs, it became apparent that the time and effort spent in discussions with the LEA was not making progress. The LEA presented an image whereby they appeared to be listening, as well as showing sympathy, but acted against the needs of Steven. In short, they were paying lip service to the actions and proceeding in their own way with what they intended to do. This is not an uncommon experience. The discussions and the panel meetings were manipulated to suit the LEA. Their interest was not Steven's individual educational needs, rather to fit him into an educational environment, which suited them.

During the interim period of the preparation of his statement, Steven attended school on a regular basis.

The school half term break had arrived and it was clear that Steven had made no further progress from when I had worked with him in Dubai. Consequently, there was a need to do the extra work with him at home, in an effort to get back on track with his learning. Steven had to be put through an intensive relearning process, which proved that he had regressed at school. It was obvious that Steven desperately needed the one-to-one support, as well as the extra Speech & Language Therapy. During this time, Steven was taught at home using the principles of ABA(Applied Behaviour Analysis). This method proved to be effective with Steven, and a video was made to demonstrate it's effectiveness to the LEA. Despite my efforts to convince the LEA of Steven's needs they did not choose to alter their view and, once again, chose to ignore Steven's needs.

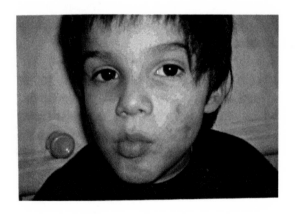

Sandy Howarth

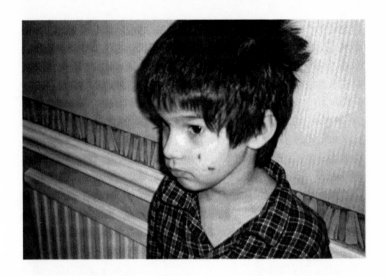

Attacks on Steven

While Steven was at school, he received scratches to his face from another child in his class. These were very deep and two years later the scars remained. Steven was also bitten through his clothes on three occasions. These five incidents in less than one year were of grave concern.

My extreme concern led me to write to the head teacher, urging a response as to what measures she was prepared to take to prevent such incidents recurring, as well as stressing the fact that these numerous attacks on Steven were a result of negligent supervision.

I note that the children demonstrating such behaviour too are ignored in the level of support they require resulting in frustrated and aggressive behaviour. Steven happened to be the child sat next to the child demonstrating aggressive behaviour through frustration.

The head teacher's response was that she did not consider her staff to be negligent, and stated that she could not guarantee the behaviour of non verbal unpredictable children, and could not expect them to behave as adults with no difficulties at all times. This response concerned me, not just for the safety of Steven, but the attitude in which the school viewed these attacks. It was my child who was the victim and I was concerned for his future if he were to remain in such an environment.

Following such a casual response, I wrote to the local mayor as well as met with the local MP. This action was taken in order to prevent further attacks as well as to gain the educational provision that Steven needed. The local MP requested answers to the relevant questions that I had raised and it was somewhat ironic that the LEA changed their view of Steven's needs and offered him a one to one support assistant. The need for extra Speech & Language Therapy was ignored.

The local Mayor, too, had questioned the school on their attitude towards the attacks and had a completely different response to that which was received by me. Their letter assured the local Mayor that they would exercise further vigilance in order to prevent such incidents recurring.

It was time for the final meeting with the LEA. The LEA was given two choices: Either to provide the extra Speech & Language Therapy that Steven needed, or to fund a full time ABA home programme. The LEA seemed to listen to all my concerns, but the outcome of the meeting was not positive. They refused the extra Speech Therapy and refused to fund a home programme, as they believed that the existing placement was satisfactory and adequate in meeting Steven's educational needs. This meeting took place at the end of the school year. Steven's support worker had been with him for one term and left at the end of her training period.

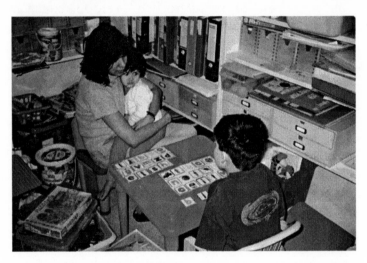

A result of a lack of choice

I felt that there was no alternative, but to withdraw Steven from school and educate him at home myself. Steven was taught at home together with his two year old sister. This was not an easy task. Nevertheless, Steven made progress which made it all worth while.

Taking the LEA to tribunal
This decision was made as an absolute last resort. After having exhausted all energies in trying to get through to the LEA as to what my child needed, and having got nowhere, meant it was time for tribunal proceedings.

Reasons for pursuing tribunal **proceedings**
My child was placed in a provision that was inappropriate
Since attending this school, Steven had been tested at home, on a regular basis, in order to find out what he had achieved at school. The results clearly indicated that there had been no progress made.

* **The LEA refused to provide the additional support that was needed**
  The continuous requests for extra Speech & Language Therapy support were ignored.
* **My child regressed due to being placed in an inappropriate setting**
  A home programme was set up, which proved that Steven had regressed in many areas during his time at school.
* **The lack of input from school meant that Steven required intensive therapy at home**
  Steven had to be taught for two hours, after school, on a daily basis. There was a significant difference in the amount of work done in two hours at the end of the day, compared with what little had been done in five and a half hours, each day at school.
* **My child was attacked**
  Steven received deep scratches to his face on two occasions and was bitten through his clothes on

three occasions during his year at an inappropriate provision.

Procedures that followed
A case was lodged at the Special Educational Needs tribunal, with all relevant documentation supporting the case.

What was included in the documentation?
* Reasons for pursuing the case against the LEA.
* Evidence of progress on the home programme.

Evidence of my child having regressed
* This was made evident by using the school's annual report compared against the parents report prepared for school, prior to Steven joining school. In addition, I provided video evidence of Steven's performance on the home programme.

Evidence of attacks
* This was shown by using enlarged colour photographs.

    Finally, the LEA was given 2 alternatives:

Option 1
* The LEA to fund the full cost of a home programme

Option 2
* The LEA to fund a place at the preferred school, together with the cost of transport, and an interim payment for the home programme till such time that Steven starts at the preferred school.

What steps did the LEA take?
The hearing was scheduled for the 14th January 2002. I received a letter close to this date from the LEA'S inspector of special educational needs. This letter requested a home visit on the 7th January 2002, to observe Steven and to assess the suitability of the home programme. Given that the visit was planned for a week prior to the scheduled tribunal hearing, led me to believe that it was planned by the LEA to gather ammunition in preparation for their tribunal representation.

The visit went very well and gave the LEA nothing to criticise. Although, there had been an urgency for the visit, I had not received a report on the observations of the programme at this point.

Time was moving closer to the scheduled hearing, when I received a voice mail congratulations message from my solicitor on the evening before the date set, stating that the LEA had conceded and agreed to fund a place for Steven at my preferred school, and fund the home programme till such time. I questioned my solicitor regarding the transport provision, and urged that he requested a part payment towards the cost of transport, to which the LEA did not agree.

I finally received the written confirmation of the LEA'S offer that had been sent to my solicitor. It had taken three weeks before I received it. Having read the letter for the first time, I was to learn that this letter had been written to mislead. It was obvious that what my solicitor led me to believe was not what was intended in the letter from the LEA.

The case had been adjourned, and I felt it necessary to meet with the Deputy for Education before a new date for the hearing was set. I met with the Deputy for Education, who studied the facts of the case, and asked the relevant questions from the LEA, with the hope that matters could be resolved. He strongly believed in my case and was rather concerned that the LEA had dug themselves a deep hole. In addition, he requested a report on the LEA's home visit, which was received 5 months late. This report had been written to criticise, but contradicted itself in its contents, which strengthened my case. Clearly, I had to be cautious about what was shown to the LEA, as there was a possibility that matters might not be resolved as expected. The matters were not resolved by discussions with the Deputy for Education, who added a great deal of pressure on the LEA, in order to prevent the case from going to tribunal. As a result, a new date for the hearing was set.

LEA's Defence
The LEA attempted to argue every point, but their defence became extremely week. Their main argument was that the home programme would cost a great deal more than the provision they had chosen for Steven. Here, again, the LEA had distorted the figures, but when the true costs were worked out, the difference didn't seem so great. The LEA chose to ignore the reasons behind my choosing to withdraw Steven from the educational setting that they chose for him, knowing very well that it wasn't an easy choice for me.

Furthermore, The LEA continuously argued that Steven's needs could be met at the provision where he regressed, and that it would be an inefficient use of resources to fund the programme that I had requested. It was obvious that the LEA had not studied the case, as they failed to recognise that Steven, having been placed in their provision and showing no progress, was a definite inefficient use of resources, which is what led me to request an alternative placement to start with.

The evidence of Steven's progress on the home programme meant that the LEA did not stand a chance at the tribunal. The new date for the hearing was 22nd April 2002. I had arrived, prepared to attend the hearing, knowing that the LEA really did not have a case. The LEA finally agreed to my requests and agreed to fund the school of my choice, with the cost of transport as well as an interim payment towards home teaching, till such time that Steven started at the new school. The case did not go to tribunal.

The LEA took me to the last hour before they conceded and agreed to my requests. In my view, it wasn't necessary to put me through all this stress and strain, but unfortunately, this is a battle that parents have to go through, so be prepared for the sake of your child. Having been through a struggle myself, I empathise with all parents who are trapped in this situation and stress the urgency in recognising your child's needs and working towards achieving the required level of support.

Steven is now 15 years of age. Having done my utmost to support Steven with his educational needs, I have recognised that the only progress he made was during the time he was taught at home by myself. It was intensive but extremely rewarding. However, allowing him to be placed in an environment, without adequate support, meant that there has been no progress made. I have retained the teaching material from the time when I last worked with Steven seven years ago, following an intensive home programme, with the hope of gaining the energy to continue that level of commitment towards teaching him. I find that Steven's time is wasted, in addition to the LEA's resources being wasted, in offering a provision which doesn't meet Steven's needs.

Education - Appropriate or inappropriate?
How would you find out if your child's educational provision is appropriate or not?

FORMS OF COMMUNICATION
Daily communication via a home school book
The school should record a summary of the day, giving details of behaviour, tasks that were worked on and how any negative behaviour was dealt with. The information from home should include events that take place during the child's time spent at home, giving details of behaviour, what leads to these behaviours and how they are dealt with, any change in diet, a lack of sleep or a change in routine.
Weekly report
This report should be a detailed report on your child's performance throughout the school week. It should include achievements on academic, physical and social skills.

Term report
A detailed report on your child's performance throughout the school term. It should cover skills that have been achieved, areas that are required to be worked on as well as targets for the next term.

The Importance of the home school book
The home school book is not only to communicate with the school but also a means of keeping a record of your child's progress. The LEA would also be able to gauge the effectiveness of the home school communication through this book. Any concerns regarding your child should be made aware to the staff working with your child via this book.

Progress chart
This can be done using a graph which will indicate if the child has progressed, plateaued or regressed. This chart can be created, using the names of skills that need to be achieved, which will give a good indication of how effective the provision is.

Do the staff working with your child understand Autism?
In many cases, staff working with your child may know little about Autism as a subject, resulting in a learning experience for them too. All members of staff should recognise and learn the complexities of Autism to enable them to deal with an Autistic child effectively. An individual, who lacks experience in dealing with Autism, could at times be harmful to your child by causing negative behaviour that could have been avoided. An Autistic child needs to trust his/her

teacher. Gaining the trust and acceptance will achieve more results when the child is ready to work.

Specialists in the field of Autism are few, but every Autistic child needs specialist help in order to learn to live a rich and happy life. They need a 100% commitment from people working with them. It is not an easy task and most give up seeing it as hard work. However, for those who have the commitment it is extremely rewarding. A person working with an Autistic child needs to learn to be alert at all times in order to avoid any upsets and minimise negative behaviour. Furthermore, the adult is required to teach the child what is acceptable or not through the use of a consistent approach.

The lack of provision and the need for additional support for Autistic children and their families has been recognised, and it is incumbent upon families to ensure that they receive the necessary support.

THE UNITED KINGDOM PARLIAMENT - DEBATE JUNE 2006

It is acknowledged that the number of cases diagnosed with Autism in the United Kingdom has risen tenfold in the past decade which has lead to a growing recognition of the support services that are of vital importance to a person on the Autistic spectrum, their families and carers.

It is acknowledged that there is no known cure for Autism but that there is much that can be done to support individuals with Autism and their families. Support services include respite, short breaks, shared care and child care.

Research has proved that trying to access services that an Autistic individual is entitled to is one of the major causes of stress affecting a family with an Autistic child. It is acknowledged that three in five families report significant levels of psychological stress. Nine out of ten had significant health needs and behavioural difficulties. It has also been noted that there could be a great deal done to reduce the levels of stress, if the needs of the family are assessed at the time of the diagnosis. However, it was evident that the many examples proved the failure to deliver such support.

An audit in 2006, of Local Authorities commissioned

by the Department of Education and Skills, stressed a need to place priority in respite services for children on the Autistic spectrum disorders. This area was picked on as an area of high importance and low availability.

It was also noted that there is strong evidence that specific family support is insufficient. The National Autistic society survey found that 70% of carers of children with Autism say that they are unable to return to work due to the lack of suitable care facilities.

Although it is recognised that short breaks are a vital part of helping families with Autism cope, 90% of short break schemes have waiting lists and children with Autism make up a third of all those on the waiting list. These services are frequently not accessible to Autistic children. The lack of availability of specialised child care is equally evident. Although, it is acknowledged that the Childcare Act will pay particular attention to the needs of disabled children, there is concern over the Local Authorities not being able to meet the demands to suit the specialist care needed by families of children with Autism to return to work.

Respite services are needed at certain crucial times, such as during holidays, but nearly all parents felt that their needs were not being met; 93% of parents did not receive help during the holidays and 87% requested a break from caring. One of the major barriers facing children with Autism is a lack of trained professionals to support them. Training is required for all relevant professionals to improve the number and quality of facilities

CHAPTER SIX

UNDERSTANDING AUTISM

Recognising your child's difficulties is vital in providing your child an opportunity to cope and move forward in life. Identifying Autistic learning, thinking and behavioural issues will assist in dealing with concerns involving your child's development. This means gaining an insight into what your child is experiencing while learning to make sense of their experience.

Parents play a key role in the bringing up of their children. In observing how parents cope with typical development, a first time parent will learn behavioural issues involving toddlers and children through trial and error. It becomes evident in typical babies that there is an inbuilt communication process in which the pitch of the cry conveys a different message. The mother learns to distinguish each cry as she learns to associate it with a particular need - an inbuilt mechanism, which is designed to protect the survival of the human species. Through this process, the parent learns to understand their child. The question is, *"how do you deal with it, when all you do doesn't seem to work or make sense?"* This is what most parents of Autistic children are faced with. The everyday rule book of bringing up children gets thrown out of the window. An inability to connect with your child, to understand their thoughts or how they are feeling, could leave a parent feeling deeply frustrated. This could result in a flood of anxiety, helplessness and even depression. The ability to connect is something that most people are wired to do. It is an occurrence in every situation where the social rules of give and take plays a role in our every day living. If this rule is not followed, we perceive that person as being rude and the rude person gradually gets isolated in society. An Autistic individual is likely to be perceived as rude by the non-Autistic population. However, if we learn to understand the symptoms associated with the condition, we could work at helping all Autistic individuals in learning to connect in the areas that they have difficulty with.

Some parents may think and feel that raising an Autistic child stops them experiencing the joys of parenthood, which isn't totally true if you step back a bit and think of who you are really feeling sad for. There is no way forward in having negative thoughts. Therefore, look at altering situations in helping and working towards a clear and effective plan for the whole family.

There are varying degrees of Autism that makes dealing with concerns different in each individual. For example, you can explain things to a child who has the ability to use language with or without the use of pictures. A child with little or no language skills can be taught through the use of pictures and basic language to support their auditory learning.

Having never had any worries or concerns of any sort prior to Steven's diagnosis of Autism, I never valued the meaning of true relaxation and peace of mind. This does not mean escaping from your responsibilities, as we all need to learn to face up to what ever life throws at us. It means looking at things in perspective while finding ways to organise the required support to enable a bright future for your child, while ensuring that he/she is receiving the best *'No matter what'* it takes to achieve it.

Autistic children display challenging behaviour due to a lack of understanding of social rules. Some of the expected challenges are screaming, aggression aimed at self, aggression aimed towards others, temper tantrums and destructive behaviour. Living with an Autistic child is a huge learning experience for any parent, not just to learn about what Autism is and about the life long impact of Autism, but to learn the true meaning of life, relationships and what is truly valuable in life.

When dealing with an Autistic child, it is important to first accept the effects that social and emotional support can provide. Without this acceptance, it will be difficult to bring out language, social or other skills. Determining the child's social and emotional age will allow you to focus on the areas of difficulty and look at obtaining further support in those areas. Identifying these needs will help towards gaining an understanding of which intervention will be most effective for the child. In order to determine the social and emotional age, it is necessary to observe the child in various situations and how they deal with each situation. A two year old can be expected to be stubborn and refuse to comply with a simple request; a five year old will engage in parallel play with peers; and an eight year old will try to model adult behaviour as they would have developed a sense of awareness of social rules and academic achievements.

An untrained carer working with an Autistic child could become confused when dealing with Autistic behaviour. The carer may place unexpected demands on the child by basing their expectations on isolated aspects of the child's abilities.

Challenging or problem behaviour is not only associated with an Autistic individual but with the non Autistic population as well. The behaviour stems from wanting to meet our own needs when faced with high levels of stress. Since Autistic individuals do not have the tools to deal with the complex and confusing world we live in an Autistic individual may deal with stress or confusion in a way that helps them release stress. It's best to nip the behaviour in the bud by recognising the early warning signs. It is necessary to recognise any build up of stress before it escalates, as it may have gone beyond control if the child is too stressed. The recognition of the underlying cause of the behaviour is crucial in tackling the situation in an effective manner, so that the child and the carer are both comfortable with the result. Each Autistic child is an individual, which will make the behaviour individual to the child's level of disability, and his/her personality. The main focus should be to find a way to communicate, in order to manage behaviour as well as to offer a sense of security to the child.

It is essential to note that people with Autism are also evolving, as they learn and absorb information through new experiences. The lack of ability to communicate may cause a barrier when gauging their level of understanding and their capacity to learn. However, given the opportunity to develop, even a non-verbal Autistic individual can reach their maximum potential. Autism itself is so complex that although the condition has its own distinct traits which are separate from other related conditions, the strength and character of each individual faced with Autism impacts further on the extent of the condition. The lack of common external traits, such as in Down Syndrome, makes it more confusing and bizarre when looking for answers. In addition, the way in which Autism is displayed in behavioural terms also varies greatly. Therefore, to understand Autism effectively and offer the required support, it is necessary to learn to see the world through the eyes of the Autistic person. Learn to enter their world and find the most effective way of understanding the condition. Being successful in recognising the world through the eyes of the Autistic person means that you will be able to offer the best possible support they need.

A child with profound learning disabilities will either be mute (and possibly use sign language) or use little communication, which is usually learnt as a response to meet his/her basic needs. In this instance, the person responsible for teaching has to input a great deal of effort in order to receive a response. For instance the child will be encouraged to say a word, the teacher will have to watch and wait for a response and if they do not receive the response, assist the child by means of prompting. The prompt should be given at the appropriate time to allow the child time to think, while preventing the child from getting overly frustrated. It is important to recognise that a scream or cry has a communicative intent as you would have from a baby, except when babyhood and toddler hood have passed it is more appropriate and acceptable to use other means of communication.

In order to be able to focus on helping an Autistic child, it is necessary that the fundamental difficulties are addressed on a psychological level. Taking a view at only the behaviour, could cause more harm and confusion and create a barrier towards helping the child make future progress. A teacher who does not understand Autism could interpret Autistic behaviour as being rude or lazy or a child with behaviour problems.

It must be noted that many Autistic children possess good rote memories, but they need a cue or prompt to recall what has been stored in their memory. In order to assist an Autistic child to think independently, it is necessary to fade away the prompts gradually, while removing the dependency on the prompts.

The Autistic mind works in a similar manner to a computer which is concrete and constant. The computer provides answers as stored on a database where it doesn't change with the spirit of things. In addition, just as computers don't have the ability to show humour, Autistic children have difficulty understanding humour. As a result, the Autistic individual becomes humorous to the normal thinking pattern of the human pack. However, unlike computers, the Autistic individual is human with feelings. Their feelings are confused due to the way in which their brains are wired. Recognition of their feelings will help towards aiding their future progress.

The individuality of Autism

Cultural behaviour in human beings is passed from one generation to the other. Some cultures cannot comprehend the thoughts or beliefs of other cultures. As a result, most human beings look for comfort in familiarity. From babyhood to toddler hood to childhood to adulthood we learn through constantly reinforcing what we have previously learnt by building on what we already know. This ability within our brain familiarises and generalises, while establishing a strength in what we already know; Based on this strength, we learn to reason and alter our thinking which enables a flexibility in understanding the thoughts of others.

An Autistic individual is not influenced by cultural beliefs. Therefore, they are not seen as part of a culture except that they fit into a group where they hold distinctive common traits. Recognising the Autistic traits together with the non-Autistic environment will help in achieving the most effective blend in bringing the two together.

Approximately 10%-15% of Autistic individuals possess above average intelligence, 25%-35% function at slightly below average intelligence or mildly affected and the remainder are profoundly affected with severe and complex needs. Most Autistic individuals show varying strengths in areas of memory, visual perception or unique talents. A successful program is one that helps an Autistic individual to use their strengths so that they learn to accept a need to fit into the particular environment.

"Help the Autistic child through allowing them to recognise a need to connect with the environment, to help overcome their difficulties while learning the skills required to function within our world"

"Offer them the support they need to achieve their best in a complex and confusing world outside their own"

Differentiating Autism

How would you know to identify a person who is Autistic and a person who isn't Autistic? Although an individual from a different country can easily be identified through their language, the way they speak, their mannerisms, their social behaviour and their style of dress, an Autistic individual who is sat quietly may not be easy to identify as being Autistic. It has been said on trips out with Steven that he didn't look like he had anything wrong. As human beings we tend to make endless assumptions. To understand Autism it is necessary to study the subject of Autism prior to making any assumptions. Many of the traits associated with Autism are also associated with other developmental disabilities such as Obsessive Compulsive Disorder, Schizoid Personality, anxiety disorders, normally developing children and ourselves. What differentiates Autism is the number of traits, the severity of the trait and the impact on the individual where it significantly impairs the ability to function.

Parents faced with challenging Autistic behaviour can quite often overlook difficult behaviour during the toddler years, which will seem as almost accepted defiance or strength of character. In this instance, it will not be too difficult for parents to face social situations as the social pressure is far less when the behaviour is accepted. I believe that the effort made at this stage is vital and will pay off as time goes on. It is a must at this stage to introduce the social rules which involve give and take, waiting and turn taking. I found that during his toddler years my Autistic child knew which buttons to push to get what he wanted, as much as other children did. A behaviour which was seeking a reaction was ignored, while behaviour which stemmed from frustration and demonstrated in an unacceptable manner meant that he needed to be removed from the situation. Children sense your lack of control in a public setting and tend to play up more, knowing their chances of having their own way through a tantrum. However, if you give in, it becomes difficult to break the pattern. Therefore, it is important to recognise from the toddler years onwards, in a child who is Autistic or not, that all challenging behaviour is a desperate need to communicate how they feel.

Parents experience moments of fatigue and powerlessness particularly in recognising or confronting challenging behaviour. A behaviour which has not been identified and dealt with at an early age leads to increased confusion resulting in escalating demands as the child gets older. The answer is to bring the parent and the child closer together through developing that all important parent child connection/bond. The importance of offering reassurance to your child at times when they are faced with a stressful situation cannot be over emphasised. Steven received constant reassurance through hugs which he resisted at first but learnt to accept once he recognised a need for it. It meant everything to me to let my child know that I felt what he felt. Having created this bond, I was able to let him know what I expected of him too. In addition, he learnt that denying him a hug meant he had done something that was not acceptable, which took away that hug. He would continuously say 'hug please' while looking for acceptance from me. I would leave him for that moment allowing him time to recognise that I wasn't pleased with his actions.

In recognising Autism, it is practical to take note of typical development and look at areas where the Autistic development is similar, lacking or vary from that of the expected process. Development from infant to adult years takes place in a sequence which is predictable at each stage of development. Typical babies are pre programmed to perform a wide range of functions within their brain and body which, through constant use, develop and expand further into adulthood. Early development involves chewing food, babbling to talking, standing to walking, controlling bladder and bowel functions, recognising and understanding space and the environment, self care and independence, to reading, writing and numerical work.

Recent research on child development has made it clear that social development is as much a pre programmed function within the brain as other psychological and physical functions. In contrast Autism is an obvious result of the lack of this pre programming which takes place in the typically developing brain. In typical development children possess the ability to recognise and generalise categories. They have the ability to place objects, shapes, people, animals and food into different categories. Furthermore, organizing and structuring our learning of different situations enables us to associate and make sense of each experience. A failure to categorize leaves each object or situation unrelated to the other, creating a disarray, which causes a barrier in putting it all into a meaningful context.

How does the Autistic individual think?
One of the main areas of difficulty that Autistic individuals are faced with is the inability to absorb information using their senses. Processing that information allows us to make sense of what has been received. Autistic learning is concrete, which indicates that words mean one thing and they are not expected to have subtle associations or added connotations. Furthermore, Autistic individuals experience challenges when faced with generalising and transferring learnt information from one situation to another. The Autistic child will try to create their own structure within their level of ability to help make sense of their world. Some possess a greater capacity to build the structure, some can do so with great difficulty, while others with a lack

of opportunity or support will experience continuous struggles throughout their lives to cope with the world, while missing out on all that life has to offer them.

Autistic individuals can learn skills and some have the ability to develop and use language, though they are unable to understand the meaning of their actions. Language is taken literally, making abstract language a puzzle to an Autistic individual. They are able to focus on detail. For example, horses being one of Steven's interests, means that he would notice an image of the tiniest horse on packaging or in a book shop from a distance or in any situation.

Autistic children tend to get easily distracted through stimulation of their own senses. Their attention could also flit from one sensation to another, be it aurally or visually. In addition, they demonstrate difficulties in differentiating and discriminating environmental sounds, leaving them overwhelmed by a bombardment of sounds and visual stimulation. Some shut out this sensory overload by preoccupying themselves with self stimulary behaviour or holding an object that may offer comfort to them.

Understanding anxiety and fears in typical development
Starting from childhood to adulthood we all experience some form of anxiety at different stages of our lives - an unpleasant sensation that results in emotional discomfort. It is a process which is accepted in young children where it is deemed as normal and an expected learning process in preparing them towards handling

unsettling and challenging situations in life.

The definition of anxiety is apprehension without cause. Although at the time that the anxiety is experienced there is no obvious threat, the person experiencing it feels that it is real and looks to escape from the situation. However, received in small doses anxiety helps us stay alert and focused. For example, fears of real life dangers help develop a sense of awareness as it enables the child to act with caution.

Anxieties and fears change throughout the developmental process from infant to adult. In babies anxiety is experienced when confronted by strangers. Toddlers show signs of anxiety when separated from their parents. Children of around four years show signs of anxiety when faced with thoughts of monsters or ghosts and children of seven years have fears of getting physically hurt.

The most typical fears in childhood development change with age although some hold onto a fear caused by an unpleasant experience. Persistent anxiety can be damaging if it takes a toll on a child's well being. In children and adults with Autism, the levels of anxiety go far beyond the levels which typical children experience and outgrow. In dealing with anxiety in Autistic children, it is necessary to be aware of the complexities of Autism as these affect the individual child.

Understanding Autistic behaviour

Autistic children pose challenges to parents and care givers due to the lack of understanding between each other. It is difficult to assess how much a non verbal Autistic child knows through watching television or information they may have acquired from their environment. A close observation of the child will help recognise the cues associated with Autistic behaviour.

Anxiety is a major factor in the life of an Autistic person. The stronger the feeling of anxiety, the more difficult it would be for an Autistic individual to cope with changes in routine or unexpected demands placed on him/her. Therefore, it is essential to identify the cause behind the anxiety and fear to find ways of dealing with the situation. The behaviours need to be dealt with through a great deal of patience, understanding and acceptance of what the child is experiencing.

Once an understanding has been established, it is necessary to find ways to resolve the behaviours while setting the boundaries in place to teach the Autistic child the meaning of acceptable behaviour. Although Autistic children respond in highly emotional ways, it is necessary to recognise that they experience a great deal of difficulty in processing their emotions which are exhibited through their confused behaviours. The ability to recall through emotional significance helps build a strong memory of an event. However, the presence of confused emotions in the Autistic person causes a barrier towards enjoying the world as the rest of us do.

"Find ways to create an enjoyable world for the Autistic child to help build on moments of happiness. Help them learn to process and recall events that they enjoy and look forward to, while offering support towards eliminating their fears."

Behaviour induced by allergies

It has been recognised that food allergies as well as dust, mould, pollen and environmental chemicals could act as triggers which cause physical and emotional problems. Above the typical allergic symptoms, they could also cause headaches, stomach-aches, bladder problems, muscle aches, sleep disorders and learning disabilities. Behaviour problems related to allergies need to be recognised early in order to help reduce any behaviour that may lead to distress, resulting in an inability to cope.

To help assess triggers in allergic reactions, keep a record of everything the child came into contact with during that day. In addition, the cause for a child developing allergies is said to be an inadequate immune system. Certain nutrients in the required amount will help strengthen the immune system.

Managing Autistic behaviour

My Programmes 1 & 2 will teach a new person dealing with your Autistic child to learn the behaviours and triggers associated with a particular situation. When working on Programme 1 follow the rules as listed.

Programme 1

Behaviour	Time/ Day	Place	Who was present?	Frequency	How was it dealt with?

- Observe the child's behaviour very closely.
- Pay attention to a pattern developing in behaviours.
- Pay attention to what sets off the behaviour and if it could have been avoided.
- Record each behaviour, reason for the behaviour, action taken and the effectiveness of the action.
- The target is to stop the behaviour from recurring. Therefore, it is extremely vital that the child is made aware of their action and why it is inappropriate.
- The adult dealing with the child must show confidence and control as well as a 100% consistency in their approach to receive a maximum level of compliance.
- Since the children displaying these behaviours have difficulty communicating how they feel, it is necessary to offer reassurance at the appropriate time.

Once you have been successful in recognising the cause for the behaviour through Programme 1, you can move on to Programme 2. This programme is to advise others of what can be done. Since the triggers can vary depending on each situation, recording as many different situations, together with temperatures and environmental factors will allow you to obtain the information required to learn to understand and deal with the child.

Programme 2

Behaviour	Cause	How was it dealt with?	Effectiveness

Dealing with Autistic behaviour
Autistic behaviour varies depending on the child's level of disability and their ability to cope.

Distress
Result of distress:
- Making inappropriate sounds.
- Crying hysterically
- Being destructive
- Directing aggression at self or others

Cause for distress:
- Confusion
- Frustration

- Difficulty with waiting
- Not having their own way

Understanding distress

In order to understand distress, it is necessary to study the child closely. Observing the child closely will enable you to learn if the child is distressed through confusion, frustration, fear or just not having his/her way.

Cause for distress
- Confusion

Behaviour
- Making inappropriate sounds

Confusion through having to accept a change in routine

A child is required to learn to deal with and accept changes in everyday life, as rigidity in routine causes a barrier in learning to live. However, to help gain the acceptance, it is necessary that the change is made clear to the child through pictures and language at the child's level. This will help the child learn to understand and cope with the situation as well as help the adult to deal with the child effectively. Routine offers security to an Autistic child encouraging learning through a predictable set of expectations. Learning flexibility in responding to different situations is an essential part of helping an Autistic child to be a part of society and the world we live in. A well structured programme with a gradual introduction to flexibility will be most beneficial for the Autistic child.

Confusion through change in teaching

Adults working with Autistic children are required to learn of issues concerning the child's level of acceptance when working with the child, while using effective methods to minimise their confusions. Although there are numerous ways of getting through to the Autistic child at his/her level, an adult who is inconsistent in their approach can do more damage than good. The adult needs to be very clear and confident when teaching, while supporting the child in accepting the change. Since most Autistic children are visually strong the support of pictures, the computer and use of videos are all effective means of easing the level of confusion. The confidence and reassurance gained from the adult will offer security to the child who resists a change in teaching.

Cause for distress
• Frustration
Behaviour
• Crying

Frustration through having to wait or take turn

An Autistic child who expresses themselves by means of inappropriate sounds, due to having to wait his/her turn, could be ignored while redirecting the attention to encourage the child to use a more acceptable means of communication. Waiting can be encouraged by means of puzzles or games supported by the use of clear and simple language - for example, 'my turn'. To encourage waiting for a longer period, a timer can be used supported by language, 'when the bell rings you can leave the table.' For children who understand completion, use the language, 'when you finish, you can go,' and for children who understand the concept of counting, 'when you count to 10 you can go.' When you are teaching waiting through counting, gradually increase the counting target to gain attention for a longer period of time. Always ensure the language is suited to the child's level of learning keeping the language simple and clear.

Frustration through having to wait in a public setting
An Autistic child may display difficulty sitting and waiting in a public space as they may feel the need to run around. In this situation it will be useful to have at hand any toys that the child is obsessed with, any favourite books, or music that the child might listen to using head phones. It would not be fair to take an Autistic child to a football match where they have no interest and expect them to keep themselves occupied. This will most definitely bring out inappropriate behaviour. In addition, they should be required to learn the concept of money, where they learn to pay for an item which is bought from a shop. Always look at the long term picture in developing life skills which are required for independent living.

Frustration through walking around a supermarket
In each situation, pay little attention to the undesirable actions while focusing on the desirable. The Autistic child can be taught to carry a basket, push a trolley, count fruit and pick up groceries as well as pay at the checkout. These skills can be taught initially through using hand on hand guidance until the child has learnt to do each task independently. Furthermore, the child

can be taught to enjoy shopping where they learn to make their own choices. The Autistic child has to learn the meaning of the word 'no' and 'put it back' from a very early age, to help teach the child that he/she cannot always have what they want.

Cause for distress
* Not being able to do as he/she wants

Behaviour
* Screaming

Distress through not being able to do as he/she wants
Autistic children must learn that life cannot always be on their terms. It is easy to give in to a tantrum. However, looking at the long term effects and working at recognising the cause will help towards managing levels of distress while gaining a social acceptance. In the event that a child displays a tantrum through not getting what they want, a firm 'no' and a quick diversion will be effective. Autistic children, like most children, will play up if they believe they can get away with unacceptable behaviour. In such circumstances, an adult who shows confidence and control will gain a maximum level of compliance from the child. Always remember that a confident approach will help your child in the long run.

Cause for distress
* Confusion

Behaviour
* Crying

Distress through confusion of departure

Autistic children feel secure with people who care for them on a regular basis and they may indicate distress when carers or parents depart. At such times, offering an explanation using language or through pictures supported by language will assist the child in understanding the departure. The child may not accept the departure in the first instance. However, allowing the child to understand the process means it's a step towards acceptance in the long term. Although it is an extremely acceptable reason for indicating distress, a child who is distressed to a level beyond control will require that the parent hold the child firmly, while reassuring the child, using a soft tone of voice: 'mummy back soon.' The adult has to have gained the confidence to know that the child will not strike out at this point, or be prepared to hold the hands before they strike. Aggression is not acceptable and has to be nipped in the bud and this method will offer the child a sense of security and assurance that he/she needs.

Anger
Cause for anger:

- Confusion with following rules
- Confusion in coping with the surrounding environment
- Escapism – refusing to comply with what is required of him/her
- Confusion in understanding what is required of him/her

Result of anger:
- Aim aggression at self
- Aim aggression at others
- Display destructive behaviour
- Aggression displayed through sounds or the use of language

Anger through confusion in coping with the surrounding

The world could be quite a bizarre and scary place for an Autistic child. He/she needs help in order to fit into this world. Therefore, it is understandable that an Autistic child expresses distress through anger in a noisy environment that is full of chaos. Bearing in mind that many people who do not display Autistic traits also experience difficulty in coping with overcrowded, closed and noisy settings, the Autistic child should be offered support to cope in this type of setting. At times when it is too much for the child to cope with, it will only be fair that the child is removed from the setting and introduced to loud noises gradually

Anger through having to work

Anger is an acceptable form of expressing feelings. However, what is not acceptable is the cause. The Autistic child must learn the meaning of working/learning to maximise their potential. Therefore, the child is required to learn strict boundaries as to when it is 'time to work' and when it is 'time to play'. This can be done through pictures, using a visual schedule to enable the child to understand what is expected of him/her, in addition to recognising an end to each task. Always start with an activity that the child enjoys, which will motivate learning while assisting towards maintaining attention for the next task.

Over excitement
Cause for over excitement:
- Being in a large open space
- Watching a favourite video
- Not having guidance and feeling out of control
- Being in a new surrounding
- An allergic reaction to food

Result of over excitement:
- Hyperactivity
- Rocking
- Flapping arms

Hyperactivity through over excitement
The behaviour of an Autistic child who becomes hyperactive through being overly excited should be assessed by the behaviour in relation to the location. Hyperactive behaviour in a park or a play ground can be acceptable to a certain extent while the child is supervised. However, behaviour which is not acceptable means that the carer is required to understand adequate methods of calming, which work for the individual child. This could involve an explanation of what the behaviour means with regard to its appropriateness, or removing the child from what is causing the hyperactive behaviour.

Rocking
The rocking movement offers comfort to Autistic children especially the individuals who indicate a

dislike to being touched or held by other people. However, rocking to music is different as it involves receiving external stimulation rather than stimulation from within themselves to a lack of apparent external influence.

Flapping arms

An Autistic child will flap his/her hands through over excitement, confusion or simply as a break from hard work. This action can be accompanied by a smile which indicates happiness or excitement. Therefore, the child should be redirected to use words to express happiness in order to fade out this behaviour, while developing an acceptable means of communication.

Attention seeking

This is a normal behaviour for children. However, when it is associated with an Autistic child it indicates a level of awareness. Although this awareness is positive, it is necessary to act on any behaviour that is inappropriate. The knowledge that this behaviour gets a reaction from others means that the child has developed a certain sense of awareness, which could also be ignored or redirected. Learn to switch off where the child recognises that the behaviour is not getting the reaction that he/she is looking for, while staying firm.

Obsessive behaviour

An Autistic child may be unusually attached to a particular object or be extremely rigid with routine, places, food, or how things are done. The reason for this behaviour is the inability to understand and cope with change. Every new experience is a learning curve which involves an effort to memorise and maintain that information in the Autistic brain. Therefore, constant changes result in an overload of disorganised information in the brain of an Autistic person. The gradual introduction to change will see a more desirable result, as the Autistic child learns to accept and organise that change within their brain to help them cope with the particular situation. An obsession, which is socially acceptable, can be used as a good motivator.

Dealing with everyday situations

In order to enjoy living as close to a normal life as possible, it is necessary to understand any setbacks, the cause and how to deal with them. Having worked with Steven over a period of time, starting from the early stages of his development, I have now found the rewards where I can enjoy a certain level of normality, as much can be expected when living with an Autistic child.

An Autistic child cannot be watched 24 hours of the day. There are times when you have to trust your instinct as well as get on with cooking or other daily chores. I have found that being on my own with two children, one Autistic, one typical, has led me to sharpen my senses. It is sometimes easier when there is just one to manage, as my daughter isn't always tolerant of her brother and may provoke a reaction that could have been avoided. However, the conflicts are rare and part of typical sibling interaction which helps Steven learn the meaning of give and take and the importance of sharing. I started a reward system for Steven's sister Riana, when she was eight years old, which I found effective, where she collected stars towards a desired item whenever she worked with her brother. Although it is generally a play based activity - for example, a 100-250 piece jigsaw puzzle, she enjoys the responsibility and the reward that comes along with it. I label the reward as: "prize awarded to Riana for earning 100 points." Working together with siblings is an effective way of encouraging joint attention, while learning to fit into and participate in groups.

Teaching your child to recognise rules
An Autistic child takes a toll on families. Therefore, it is necessary that they do not feel that life is all on their own terms. As much as rewarding positive behaviour is a crucial part in the early stages of teaching an Autistic child, they must learn that life is not about constant rewards, be it social, a food item or a toy. The Autistic child must be taught to accept that there are disappointments in life too, and that they cannot always get what they want. The way to develop a level of acceptance is by building a trust, where the child learns to understand and feel comfortable in our world. The child comes out of their world and into our world where they become more tolerant of what is expected in the non-Autistic world. Do not push expectations too early. A gradual introduction to new situations is a valuable part of integrating an Autistic child into society. I have learnt through a consistent approach that as much as it is easy to give in, ignoring works very well too. Once you gain the strength to not let the behaviour get to you, is the time when you have accomplished a major breakthrough in dealing with challenging behaviours. You will recognise that the Autistic child who is in

their own world will come out of their world when it is something they really want. They will read your facial expression, your verbal response or your lack of response. For example, my son makes constant eye contact when it means something that he wants. After having said no, I ignore him. I am only able to do this since I have learnt the strength to let him understand that I make the rules and not him. This in turn works well with my daughter as she recognises a certain level of fairness in our everyday family life. An inconsistent approach in dealing with behaviours allows the Autistic child to believe that the stronger the negative behaviour the more likely it is that you will give in and let them have their own way.

Creating a bedtime routine

Many children with Autism experience difficult or erratic sleep patterns where their brain has difficulty in recognising when to wind down and when to switch off. Some stay awake for hours, some go to bed very late at night when they choose to do so, while others leap about getting hyperactive. Getting Steven into a bed time routine was quite a task. However, developing a regular routine helped reduce the wakeful nights, where they gradually became less frequent and finally paid off in many ways. We do have the odd disturbed night but he has learnt the routine, in that on occasion when he does have a wakeful night he has learnt that he is expected to remain in bed. The bed time routine was established through a strict and consistent approach. First Steven was taught that at 7pm it was time for his bath followed by getting dressed into his pyjamas, followed by a warm mug of milk at 7.30pm, after which he was given half an hour to unwind and at 8pm it was time for him to use the toilet, wash his face and brush his teeth. He was taken to bed immediately after, where he was given some books to look at while listening to relaxing music. At 8.30pm it was lights out and time to sleep. It is a relief to say that I don't have to stay up listening out for Steven at night, and I too am able to enjoy a good night's sleep. It may be a battle of wills at first but it is necessary to be strict and consistent in order for it to work. We are all less tired. The lack of sleep could result in confused or aggressive outbursts resulting in upsetting the rest of the family in destroying their strength to function normally. This routine also helps when going away, be it on holiday or even a weekend away. Through years of difficulty, from babyhood till he was around six years of age, Steven has now learnt the sleep time routine well. In addition, he understands flexibility when the bed time routine is a little delayed for some reason or other, while at times he would take himself to bed.

Time out
A positive and effective way of dealing with behaviour which allows the child to calm down by removing them from the situation that brought out the negative behaviour. The child needs to understand very clearly through pictures, symbols, words or stories - whichever is suited to the child's level of understanding - that the time out is given for a reason and what that reason is. The complete process should also be explained as the purpose behind the approach is to minimise and eliminate the behaviour. The time out method is one that I used with Steven at times when the behaviour

resulted in aggressive outbursts, where he hurt his sister, only due to not having his own way. I have learnt to predict a likelihood of the behaviour escalating by using the method to prevent any further aggression. In following the time out method, removing the child from the situation gives the child time to calm down. The child will be taken into a separate room where he/she cannot hurt them self, which can be constantly monitored. A few minutes is all that may be required. In dealing with Steven, I would stand outside and ask "Steven are you calm now?" to which he would repeat rather than reply as being rote leant "I am calm now". I would let him out of the time out room, while observing his reactions and letting him learn that the first instance he attempted to raise his hand to strike out, that he would be taken straight back in for more time out.

Redirecting negative behaviour

Redirecting the attention from a situation that could cause distress will be an effective approach in minimising any undesirable behaviour. At times a reaction can be inevitable, especially on occasions when it involves siblings and their needs or in social situations. At such times, it is best to be prepared with a distracter that could work to diffuse the situation. It should be something that the child finds satisfaction in, which is not at hand on a regular basis. In this instance, action has been taken in predicting the behaviour, while finding a suitable solution to prevent the situation from getting out of control.

Helping an Autistic individual to understand and cope with their feelings

Autistic individuals display difficulty in managing their feelings. They exhibit confusion and distress as a result of an inability to cope with how they feel. Familiarising themselves with their own emotions allows the individual to develop an awareness of how they feel, while learning to cope with their feelings. Furthermore, the frustration of an inability to process one's own feelings causes a great deal of confusion which leads to anxiety and results in unacceptable behaviour. Teaching an Autistic child facial expression and body awareness in themselves, as well as in others, using as many situations to help explain the associated meaning of each expression, will help reinforce their knowledge of the complexity of feelings.

In developing awareness of feelings in Steven, I started by creating six images indicating the basic feelings: happy, sad, scared, angry, sleepy and tired. The cards were individually laminated and stuck onto a further laminated card, using Velcro tabs. Steven was observed while paying attention to his mood and acting on opportunities when he expressed distress, joy or how he felt. The picture relating to how he felt was removed and held up to him at each point together with the prompt - for example, 'I am happy', 'I am angry', 'I am sleepy', 'I am scared', 'I am tired' or 'I am sad'. These were taught using the pictures together with facial expressions and body language. Furthermore, we worked on additional feelings such as hot and cold, ill, sick, hurt, (as in physical pain) itchy, hungry and thirsty. Teaching the meaning of these feelings offers security as well as confidence to the Autistic individual, letting them know that you understand how they feel.

At times, when the levels of anxiety leads to distress, effective methods of calming can be used to soothe and relax the child – for example, a warm bath, music, a massage or redirecting the child to an activity that they enjoy. Autistic children also calm themselves and enjoy the motion of a swing or a jump on a trampoline. Anxiety, when expressed through anger and aggression, should be dealt with in a similar manner to dealing with any other aggression. However, the adult will be required to offer assurance at the appropriate time, to allow the child to recognise your awareness of their feelings. Ensure the child has calmed completely prior to offering any form of comfort, or it could be recognised as rewarding inappropriate behaviour which is not the aim of the behaviour management plan. Dealing with such behaviour takes a bit more confidence and control as the child has to recognise that you understand how they feel but that they are not allowed to strike out or show any aggressive behaviour. The child should be allowed to calm down in their own time. Such behaviours emphasise the significance in developing a means of communication to help express their feelings through distress or joy, in addition to learning to request their needs.

Uta Frith explains that the difficulties displayed by Autistic individuals which result in loneliness are due to more than just an inability to express and understand emotion, but also to a difficulty in knowing and believing. The complexities of the world become apparent when you begin to wonder if your child knows to differentiate between reality and fantasy. Is the world of fantasy created by Disney real to the Autistic child?

Understanding and treating self injurious behaviour

An Autistic child who displays self injurious behaviour can be most devastating to any family. Forms of the behaviour include head banging, hand biting, excessive rubbing of the skin or scratching. Collecting data on the behaviours will help explain the causes behind the actions. Data should be collected on the type of behaviour, frequency, duration, severity of the behaviour, physical and social environment, lighting, sounds, any person who was present at the time, time of day and day of the week.

Researchers have learnt that levels of certain neurotransmitters are associated with self injurious behaviour, where self injury increases the production of Beta-endorphins or the release of endorphins, which in turn is said to result in the individual experiencing an anesthesia - like feeling, which shuts off pain while engaging in the behaviour. The child learns to enjoy the feeling, while not recognising the pain or injury that is caused by it. If the result of injury is biochemical, there may not be a relation to the individual's environment and injury, where a biochemical approach will be required in combating the symptoms.

Behaviour management rules

The key to successful behaviour management is consistency. Giving in to unacceptable behaviour as a matter of convenience or to avoid a scene in public is an easy option. However, behaviours which are dealt with in a manner where any negativity is recognised early enough to nip it in the bud, will result in an easier to manage child as time goes on. Learn to switch off any thoughts of who is present at the time as a child will sense a weakness or lack of control and the child will play on it to get his/her own way. Behaviour which is harmful to the child or others has to be recognised and dealt with immediately. However, harmless, self stimulary behaviour that is not likely to upset anyone means that you have the choice to allow it as a trait in the child. Harmless behaviour that invites a negative reaction from the public - for instance, leading to the child being picked on, may be better to be redirected to a socially more acceptable behaviour. The sole purpose behind the plan is for the benefit of your child and his/her future. The long term goal should be aimed at acceptable behaviour, be it living and working together with others or alongside others.

How do Non Autistic peers see Autistic behaviour?

Autistic behaviour will be seen as odd and bizarre by their non Autistic peers even at times when the child possesses language. An Autistic child's interests are not social rather self directed or related to objects. They lack any motivation to interact with their peers and spend time engaged in obsessive or solitary play.

EARLY SIGNS OF BEHAVIOUR IN "TYPICAL" / "AUTISTIC" DEVELOPMENT

Typical development
In typical development, children develop through a predictable set of skills during a predictable time frame. These skills are referred to as development milestones, which are assessed through gross and fine motor skills, speech and language skills, independence skills and social and emotional development. Failure to achieve these milestones at the expected time results in developmental delay. Development in each area influences the development in other areas; for example, the development of speech and language influences social and emotional development.

Attachment, sharing interests or feelings
Behaviour in early childhood indicates a strong attachment to parents and carers. The child will remain close to or in the vicinity of the adult while constantly checking to ensure that the adult is still around. They look at ways to interact as they recognise and learn to enjoy the attention. Autistic children demonstrate over attachment when a parent or carer leaves a home setting and a lack of attachment to the parents or carers when they are out in public. Here the type of attachment in an Autistic child tends to contradict itself as they show a desperate need to control what is familiar to them in one situation but not in another. The lack of attachment to carers in a public setting indicates a lack of awareness to danger combined with an attachment, which is on their terms. Unlike in typically developing children, the Autistic child will not look back once they

181

wander off. A sign of social isolation is at social events, when the Autistic child looks for ways to spend time away from others to be on their own. I recognised social withdrawal in Steven when he was 2½ years old. He enjoyed his paddling pool a great deal though at times, when other children got in at the same time as him, he would choose to get out and walk away. In recognising the Autistic behaviour, I resolved it very early by insisting that he stayed in with the other children. This resulted in a great deal of protest to start with - but was necessary in teaching Steven to accept other children in play as well as socially. In learning to accept other children, Steven learnt flexibility in adapting to a world outside his own.

Eye Contact
Early development in babies and toddlers demonstrate a constant use of eye contact. During the early years, babies and toddlers use eye contact as a means of bonding and seeking reassurance from parents while learning to recognise their boundaries as they get older.

Autistic Development
Lack of sharing interests
Sharing their toddler's interests and playing with them at their level is an enjoyable moment for any parent. The interaction of an Autistic child could be a tickle that they enjoy and at most times, their interests will be seen as focused solely on themselves. Early interaction in Steven indicated times when he constantly carried a book with torn pages or a broken toy to his dad's hands. He would give it to his dad's hands, avoiding eye contact with his dad, while expecting the pages to be

taped together or the broken toy to be fixed. This lack of social awareness indicates the Autistic child uses adults as tools. These are the hands that fix, feed or give them what they need. I used these moments as opportunities to develop eye contact, although Steven does still need to be reminded to look when requesting a need, he doesn't feel threatened by eye contact or the proximity of others.

A normally developing child will use repeated facial expression in an effort to make known to the adult their feelings, preferences or dislikes. For example, my daughter Riana was particularly expressive at five months old. She sat on her high chair tasting different varieties of fruit which were on the plate in front of her. She tasted a segment of tangerine and made an expressive face which suggested that what she had tasted was sour. Here she didn't only taste the fruit but also communicated her knowledge of the taste. Following a reaction, she repeated the action over and over again using facial expressions while chuckling and kicking her feet at the same time. This is a typical sense of interaction and sharing joy.

Leading an adult by the hand
An Autistic child will take your hand to something he/she wants. The child may clasp an adult's hand without the use of eye contact. This is a typically Autistic trait in non verbal children. The majority of normally developing toddlers will point and babble along with using continuous eye contact to compensate for the lack of verbal language, as opposed to just leading an adult by the hand. Steven led an adult by the

hand starting from around the age of 2 years and at one point Steven was even prepared to walk away with a stranger. In this instance, the adult had a similar build and style of clothing to his dad. He took the adult for a walk around the garden, at a social gathering. Following the walk, they both returned and the adult who knew of Steven's Autism was moved by the thought that he had been chosen by Steven to go for a walk. However, it was clear once Steven returned, heard his dad's voice and looked up at his dad that he realised he had gone for a walk with the wrong person.

Lack of imitation

During the early stages of development, babies and toddlers copy much of what they see, while learning to imitate without any encouragement. Early imitation is seen as a way that babies process information non verbally, which takes place through play, through objects and through using their body. An Autistic child, who lacks interest or awareness of others, fails to see a need to imitate and as a result, the ability to imitate has to be taught.

Lack of understanding the feelings of others

An Autistic child will demonstrate great difficulty in coping with our world. Our world consists of dealing with other humans as well as our selves. The lack of awareness of how others feel is a major factor in Autism, which causes a barrier when living in our world. A person who is not trained in Autism will find the lack of understanding of facial expressions, vocal intonation and emotion in language rather tiresome to deal with. A normally developing child will offer comfort in their own way to someone they see as being in distress. They may offer a hug, a favourite toy or share a sweet. The Autistic child does not show awareness of emotion. For example, Steven indicated a lack of awareness of emotion in others while watching his crying baby sister. Although he showed a great deal of attachment to his sister, he would say "waaa aaa babee" The same as he would say "dog woof woof". Steven called his sister "babee" during her early years. Though, he now calls her both her name and "babee" at different times. The world perceives a person who lacks emotion and feeling as being cold hearted. This is not true when referring to a person with Autism. The difficulty in recognising and processing their own feelings explains why they cannot cope beyond themselves.

Unusual language development
Autistic children who do speak often use language in unusual ways. Some retain parts of early stages of their language development; some speak in single words. Some repeat phrases over and over again or repeat what they hear. This is called echolalia. For instance, if you ask the question "what do you want" an Autistic child may repeat "what do you want".

Lack of attention
The attention span of an Autistic child is at its best when the child is interested in the activity. To gain attention in the areas outside the child's own interests is a task in itself. The Autistic child does not show interest in becoming independent and will be content in allowing an adult to dress them or deal with other self

care tasks.

Interaction with adults

Interaction with adults was a great deal easier for Steven as he knew that he could use them to get what he wanted. Steven received a positive response from adults due to his good looks. On one particular occasion when Steven was around 10 years old, during a visit to Kensington Park I sat with Riana watching him while giving him space to explore his surroundings. I thought he would enjoy this time on his own but to my surprise, I found him sat on the lap of one of two eighteen year old girls. I ran over to the girls to apologise and explain his Autism. The girls thought he was lovely and were happy to let him stay with them as we sat beside them. Steven chose to sit on the lap of the heavier girl who had the more comfortable lap. I recognised it from a previous occasion when he chose to sit on a strangers lap at a party who too was overweight.

As Steven reached his teenage years, he seemed to have developed more awareness where he has recognised the need to stay together as a group. This has made my life easier. In addition, Steven has learnt a certain level of independence as he doesn't require an adult to hold his hand at all times. On one occasion, while walking with Riana and myself, Steven decided that he wanted some sweets and stopped at the sweet shop and refused to move when he was asked to keep walking. We continued to walk and Riana was concerned that Steven was left behind. When he realised that he couldn't get what he wanted and that he could lose us, he hurried to catch us up. This level of compliance was developed through letting Steven learn from a very early age that life wasn't on his terms.

SYMPTOMS RELATED TO AUTISM
Repetitive behaviour
A behaviour that sets the Autistic child apart from other normally developing children. Although the Autistic child may appear physically normal they tend to display behaviours such as arm flapping, wiggling toes, sudden freeze in position, constant spinning and repetitive play.

Resistance to change
An Autistic trait where the child recognises something insignificant to the rest of us as causing a great deal of distress to themselves in the event that item is changed or moved. Consequently, this rigid behaviour pattern causes exploring new surroundings or new routes to places tiresome for some parents. Therefore, it is necessary to recognise the cause for distress. The Autistic child has great difficulty understanding and coping with the world we all perceive so naturally. Support them in retaining that order while introducing gradual changes in routes.

The developmental paediatrician who first assessed Steven, explained Autism to us in a way that I found to be very clear and explicit. He described the Autistic brain as similar to lacking a scaffolding as opposed to the normally developing brain, which had an inbuilt frame in place. When information is obtained from the environment, it is automatically placed on the scaffolding in relation to where it belonged and can be recalled, transferred and added onto at any time. Each time a child sees something familiar, it reinforces the knowledge and builds upon that knowledge. He said that the Autistic child had to build the scaffolding from scratch as well as place every bit of information on the frame in the place where it belonged. Without the scaffolding the information floats around while causing the world to be an even more bizarre and confusing place. An Autistic child needs help to build the frame to make sense of the world. This explains the reason behind an Autistic child's desire to hold onto what they already know, while resisting change. It is comforting and helps them feel secure. In addition, it is information they gathered through great difficulty in building their own framework.

A visual schedule which incorporates pictures of the activities that have been planned for the day and the sequence of events that are to take place will assist in adjusting to a change. A visual schedule which is prepared for each child should be thought out clearly to suit the child's level of learning. A structured day offers security to Autistic children. Therefore, a gradual process, using the most suited method of communication for the individual child, will minimise confusion and gain acceptance from the Autistic child in entering our world.

Self stimulary behaviour
A pattern of behaviour which is displayed by most Autistic children. The signs of self stimulary behaviour are evident from an early stage in life where the emergence of language helps reduce and eliminate the symptoms in some children, and in others it continues

into adulthood. Behaviours include flapping arms, walking on tip toes, rocking, head banging and spinning.

Head banging

Head banging is associated with frustration. Steven head banged on a regular basis from 15 months up until 2½ years of age. However, he made it a point to place a cushion on the hard floor prior to banging his head on it. On one occasion he placed the cushion on me while I had turned my back to him to do the dishes and banged his head on the cushion. Although this behaviour stopped by the age of four years when he was worked with at home, it has reoccurred on occasion due to a lack of provision at school which has resulted in frustration in communicating his needs.

Learning your child is Autistic

To learn that your perfectly healthy looking baby is Autistic is something that any parent would find difficulty in dealing with. The first feeling is shock, followed by the realisation of the life long condition which devastates most parents. Most parents look at ways of coping while each copes according to what suits them best taking into account their strengths and weaknesses.

I coped with the Autism by first shutting myself out, to give me time to think things through. I did not go into denial but accepted it and shutting myself out gave me time to grieve and look at what could be done to help my son. During the grieving process, I didn't truly know where to start or what could be done to help my son. Going into denial is a natural way of coping with emotional trauma. However, I felt that it meant I was not accepting Steven for who he was. It was a shock, that day after day I felt a sense of numbness within me. I looked forward to going to bed at night and hoped that when I woke up the Autism would be gone. I observed Steven at every opportunity and I tried to see the good in him. He was happy at most times, which was good, but this meant he was happy being in his own world, while the rest had to be worked on. The grieving and learning period took months but once I knew what to do I decided to teach Steven myself.

CONDITIONS ASSOCIATED WITH AUTISM

Mental retardation

Although it has been said that a high proportion of individuals with Autism suffer from mental retardation, research studies have been inconclusive. Verbal IQ tests that have been carried out on nonverbal children have resulted in an inaccurate estimate of the child's level of intelligence. A 'Test Of Nonverbal Intelligence' (TONI) will be more accurate in gauging the child's level of ability. The result of any intelligence test is only to assess the level while therapy and education will help meet the child's needs.

Seizures

It has been estimated that 25% of Autistic individuals, some in early childhood and others in adolescence, develop seizures. Changes in hormone levels are said to be likely to trigger seizures. Seizures range from mild, which can be noticed as a gaze or absent spell for a few seconds, to severe, grand mal seizures. Many Autistic individuals are said to have sub clinical seizures that may go unnoticed but can have a drastic effect on mental ability. Results of tests suggest that a short EEG, which takes around one to two hours, will not be able to detect any abnormal activity. Therefore, a twenty four hour EEG may be necessary. There are drugs used for the treatment of seizures. However, these could have harmful side effects, which mean the child's health needs to be checked on a regular basis.

CHAPTER SEVEN

PERVASIVE DEVELOPMENTAL DISORDER

Autism fits within the umbrella of Pervasive Developmental Disorder which covers five disorders. The most recognised is Autism, though Rett Syndrome, Childhood Disintegrative Disorder, Asperger's Syndrome and Pervasive Developmental Disorder Not Otherwise Specified are the remaining four disorders. Although PDD children and Autistic children can display similar symptoms and common difficulties, each child carries his/her own individual personality.

- *Autism*
- *Asperger's Syndrome*
- *Rett Syndrome*
- *Childhood Disintegrative Disorder (CDD)*
- *Pervasive Developmental Disorder Not Otherwise Specified (PDD-NOS)*

Asperger's Syndrome
A condition which takes longer to detect problems, as a child affected by Asperger's Syndrome may not indicate or may show only limited difficulties in language development. The time when a parent takes note of the condition and expresses concern is when they notice oddness in social behaviour, language or the manner in which they choose to play. These children are very rarely mentally retarded while being generally seen as odd with unusual interests. Children with Aspergers may not receive the support they need as it isn't officially recognised as a condition that involves a

learning disability. Their interests and signs of oddness tend to have them playing on their own at most times. It is said that these children have been known to have been subjected to bullying. This is an area which should be addressed from an early age to assist the child in building their self esteem, by removing the barrier in developing social skills.

Individuals with Aspergers Syndrome are socially awkward, which results in a difficulty to make friends. The failure to create lasting social relationships is the lack of ability to reciprocate. The "give and take" in a normal relationship. The conversations are self centred and show a lack of interest in others. Furthermore, Aspergers individuals express difficulty in making social decisions, while lacking a sense of awareness in recognising social cues through general observations of others and situations.

Aspergers children who are not diagnosed at an early age, who don't receive the help they need, grow up feeling isolated. They recognise that they are different to their peers but cannot understand why they are different. As with Autism, children with Aspergers need to be recognised, accepted and supported in order to help them cope with their difficulties.

Rett Syndrome
A rare disorder, which affects mostly females. They start by showing normal development and move onto displaying Autistic like symptoms between 6-18 months. They lose their abilities in the use of language, social development, and the ability to control their feet.

A most noticeable trait of Rett Syndrome is the wringing movement of the hands. In addition, children with this condition have the potential to lose their mobility as well as develop severe mental retardation. Treatments are used to help with problems related to co-ordination speech and movement. These include physiotherapy, and Speech Therapy. Furthermore, though the condition has been recognised as one of the five PDDs, scientists have indicated that the Rett Syndrome is a separate developmental disorder and not a part of the Autistic spectrum.

Childhood Disintegrative Disorder
A disorder in which children develop normally until they are 2 years old. Signs of the condition appears between 3 and 4 years of age when the child loses previously acquired skills in intellectual, social and language development. The longer period of normal development sets the diagnosis of CDD apart from Rett Syndrome.

Pervasive Developmental Disorder Not-Otherwise Specified (PDD-NOS)
The term given to a person who indicates impairments in social interaction, communication and stereotyped behaviour, but does not fit into the other four pervasive developmental disorders.

OTHER CONDITIONS THAT COULD BE CONFUSED WITH AUTISM

- *Fragile X Syndrome*
- *Severe hearing impairments*
- *Severe visual impairments*
- *Developmental language disorder*
- *Semantic-Pragmatic Disorder*
- *Elective mutism*
- *Socially deprived child*
- *Attention Deficit Disorder*

Fragile X Syndrome

The most common form of genetically inherited mental retardation. A blood test is carried out to determine the presence of a fragile area in the chromosome. The mother as the carrier passes the disorder on to her sons. Males carry a single X chromosome and a single Y chromosome while females have two X chromosomes. Girls are less affected as the extra chromosome can be used instead of the faulty one. Children with Fragile X have recognisable physical features that are associated with the condition. These children are seen as odd but friendly and sociable. Characteristics include high arched pallet, strabismus (lazy eye), large cupped ears, flexible joints (double jointed), poor muscle tone, flat feet, sometimes heart valve abnormalities and longish faces. In addition to recommended treatments to assist in behaviour problems, Speech & Language disorders and sensory impairments, families are advised to seek genetic counselling to understand the inherited nature and the likelihood of the condition being passed onto future offspring.

Severe hearing impairments

Children with hearing impairments display signs of learning difficulties associated with language. These difficulties result in behaviours as seen with Autism. They are different to Autistic children as they prove their ability to form social relationships, use gestures, show facial expression, mime, use sign language and use their imagination.

Autism can be sometimes associated with deafness. To differentiate one from the other, it is vital to recognise the associated behaviours through responses to sounds, music and videos. An Autistic child will show awareness or sensitivity to certain sounds while ignoring other sounds. A deaf child will demonstrate an equal lack of awareness to most sounds.

Severe visual impairment

Children who display visual impairments demonstrate signs of Autistic behaviour such as stereotyped movements. This is likely to be a result of the lack of visual stimulation from the environment.

Developmental language disorder

Children with developmental language disorders show difficulty with receptive and expressive language. Receptive being the ability to understand language and expressive being the ability to use language. A child who is unable to use expressive language will require help in bringing out the sounds and learning to form and articulate the sounds. Children who lack the ability to gain speech will use gestures, facial expressions and sign language as a means of communication. Children who learn to read and write can use this skill to communicate not just their needs but at a social level, which will enable them to gain further opportunities in realising their potential.

Semantic-Pragmatic Disorder

A child with a disorder in which they are capable of using speech but indicate a great deal of difficulty in understanding speech. They use repetition as a means of trying to understand what is being said. These children have good memories and have the ability to learn to read, but have difficulty comprehending what they read.

Elective mutism

A disorder in which the child speaks only in one situation. They may speak in a familiar environment such as home but stay silent in every other situation. This disorder can be associated with other developmental disorders as well as Autism.

Socially deprived child

A baby who is deprived of affection, warmth and stimulation from the environment is likely to fall behind in their development. They will display signs of backwardness in their social, language and intellectual development. The withdrawn nature of these children could resemble Autism. However, the socially deprived child is different to the Autistic child in that the child has the ability to function as normally developing children do, once he/she receives the care and stimulation that was initially lacking.

Attention Deficit Disorder
Children and adults with attention disorders tend to get easily distracted or drift away into their own worlds. This could cause a barrier towards effective learning. However, a disorder which lacks any accompanying behavioural issues could easily go undetected and undiagnosed leaving the child or adult missing out on the opportunity to receive the additional support they require. At times when Attention Deficit Disorder is accompanied by hyperactivity, the child tends to act impulsively and show a lack of ability to sit still or wait to take their turn. Parents are left drained of their energy and teachers feel that the class is often disrupted. As adults, they have difficulty in organising themselves and completing tasks to listening and following directions.

Autism - The groups
Autistic children fit into different categories depending on their personalities, and abilities.

- *The aloof group*
- *The active but odd group*
- *The stilted group*
- *The passive group*

The aloof group
Autistic children who fit into this group do not respond to their name or if you were to try and make conversation with them. They look past you and pull away if you try to hug them, and do not show expression except for when they are extremely angry or extremely excited. They respond to being tickled, or

swung around.

The active but odd group

These children are seen as physically active and able to speak. They will actively approach an adult but only to express their needs. They lack interest in the feelings of others. The eye contact too is odd rather than lacking as they may stare long and hard at the person they are talking to making it appear as though they are talking at the person. Although these children approach people a lack of social understanding means that, they have difficulty interacting in an appropriate manner.

The over-formal, stilted group

This group of Autistic children are considered the most able of the groups. Any disability may only be recognised as the child gets older or even moves onto adulthood. They are extremely well mannered and very well behaved, making them socially accepted. Although they lack social understanding, they work hard at learning social rules and what is expected. This lack of understanding makes it difficult for them to learn to adapt from one situation to the other. As in most Autistic children, they have difficulty understanding the thoughts and feelings of others.

The passive group

Children in this group are quiet and tolerant. They display less behavioural problems and accept social interaction, but they will not initiate it.

CHAPTER EIGHT

PARENTS' CONCERNS

Parents are faced with an array of concerns when dealing with an Autistic child. Reaching out for what the future holds while struggling to obtain services becomes a priority. Nevertheless, a positive future for an Autistic child is one that offers them the support to achieve their full potential. The opportunity to gain meaningful language offers greater promise for an Autistic child who can use language to communicate and cope within our world. However, a child who demonstrates passive behaviour has a greater potential to learn through their level of acceptance and tolerance in situations as a rule. In addition a general compliance with learning will enable more people to work with the child allowing the child the opportunity to acquire more skills, which will create a positive impact on the child's future.

A greater awareness of Autism and special needs today has resulted in an increase in acceptance from society and services than previously recognised. The interventions that have been recognised as treatments for Autism suggest that there is a great deal more hope than it was previously thought possible. However, when it comes to obtaining services the children with less severe symptoms who are more able to adapt tend to benefit most. Added learning difficulties and profound and complex needs means extra resources which I have found through experience are not readily available. This leaves the Autistic child with a greater need for support struggling further as the years go by. The struggle that parents are faced with is that a demanding Autistic child exhibits a strength of character in expressing their level of frustration in dealing with the world. However, the authorities choose to ignore the strength while seeing it as a difficult or no hope situation. This is a totally narrow minded view.

Severely affected children who do not receive adequate support tend to be less likely to live independently. Though, children who gain the ability to integrate stand a greater chance in living independently as adults. Though, it is said to be rare as most Autistic individuals have shown a need for some degree of supervision as they reached adulthood.

Concerns and stress on family
A child who lacks meaningful play and social interaction is a cause for concern to most parents. A child may display unpredictable behaviour or be a danger to themselves or others or even considered a nuisance to those who may not be so tolerant. As a result parents feel a need to watch their child constantly. The behaviours tend to take time away from time to relax which leaves a parent overly tired and drained of energy to function normally on a daily basis. It is a must that parents find time to relax and function within a family setting. Finding the most effective ways of dealing with situations will help eliminate the stress levels which stop a family from functioning normally.

Most children make friends easily as they are able to interact socially or occupy themselves. An Autistic child who lacks leisure skills needs a constantly structured and supervised day which makes the flexibility of family life, social events and holidays tiresome. The additional challenges of getting their child off to sleep keeps the parents drained of all energy. Letting it reach this stage is harmful to the parents as well as to the rest of the family. A parent in such a situation is likely to end up suffering from burnout, depression or other health problems.

Dealing with health issues and the role of caring
A further issue that parents are faced with is when leaving an Autistic child with a carer other than themselves to have a break. Steven is now a teenager and attends an Autistic day school. However, when he returns home from school, he expects me to be with him at all times. I have been with him nearly all of his life except on two occasions when it was absolutely necessary to be away from him. The first instance was a two day stay in hospital when my daughter was born in March 1999 and the second in August 2004 again a trip to hospital but this time to have a hysterectomy. The thoughts and concerns of how Steven would be cared for left me suffering for two years prior to reaching a decision to finally have my health sorted. The point at which I felt the need was when the lack of energy impacted on my ability to cope. I managed to get the required help in place while informing all concerned in caring for the children that I was on the end of a phone line.

Once the care for the children was arranged I learnt to relax. I was expected to arrive a day early at the hospital to allow me to rest as well as prepare for the operation. The surgeon and his team visited me the previous evening to explain the procedures and questioned me on the sort of help I had in place. Although, I did have help in place it wasn't enough to help me through the recovery process. I replied that I had hoped to bounce back to which the surgeon replied 'you won't'. I needed to know how much I could do once I returned home to which I was told that all I could do was to get up from bed and walk to the couch. Although, I didn't want to believe it to be true, it was.

At this point the hospital staff spoke to Steven's social worker requesting support for when I returned home and urged that it was granted as a matter of urgency. In addition I was given two extra days in hospital as being a sole carer for an Autistic child.

I was advised by the hospital specialists to take it easy and not carry children or do any heavy work. Going into hospital to have a hysterectomy was such a lovely holiday and I really enjoyed it. Returning home although I had help with the children for part of the day, I was alone with the children at night, I found myself completely forgetting my stitches and rushing over to Steven, on the first night, when he played up and became hyperactive through all the confusion. Thinking positively having Steven helped me recover and heal faster than I had expected. Having the help as well as not being able to function as efficiently as I normally would have, taught to me to relax. I learnt that getting stressed was the last place I ever wanted to be, and I have since tried to do as much as possible to keep myself healthy.

I recall having to shuffle to move from place to place which got me quite impatient to recover. Going out on my own for the first time meant, crossing at the pedestrian crossing before the lights changed. I found that drivers made allowances for the elderly crossing the road but seemed to toot impatiently, when I was crossing as they couldn't see an obvious problem. It took six weeks to three months before I could start functioning normally and a year to feel completely back to normal. I feel that sorting my health has given me a new energy that I am now able to run rather than having to resort to shuffling.

Organising respite care

Many parents end up not going out due to the difficulties in finding people who can deal with an Autistic child. Parents stay in where turning down invitations develops into a habit, which leads to people automatically leaving you out while assuming that you are unable to leave your Autistic child. In an effort to avoid any setbacks at home, I chose to stay in over the years as I believed that it was easier to stay in than to worry about a person's ability to deal with Steven without causing him distress.

My time away in hospital in August 2004, through need, expressed an urgency and informed me of the importance of introducing Steven to other people. However, it always seemed like too much effort to even contemplate arranging respite care. Having had many ups and downs during the past year, in recognising situations with regard to Steven, I decided to make a conscious effort in getting out and having a break myself. My primary focus was to teach Steven to accept other people a part from myself. It was a strain at first even resulting in aggressive outbursts, where Steven clearly expressed his level of distress. To enable him to feel secure with the new situation I created a visual board to explain each step of the process. The pictures explained each step which was to take place, starting with my going out, Steven staying with the child minder and his sister, going to sleep at bed time and my returning home. To begin with it proved to be a tiresome process as Steven refused to accept any new person. However, four months on he has learnt to accept the change where I now feel assured by the availability of people who are willing and capable of dealing with Steven. A slow process but again it is a vital step towards helping your child learn flexibility in accepting new people and adjusting to change.

Coping with anger and disappointment
Dealing with an Autistic child could cause a great deal of stress resulting in an inability to cope. This in turn leads to depression and anxiety which takes a toll on the mother and the Autistic child as well as the rest of the family. It is quite natural to feel anger or disappointment as dealing with the word Autism alone is a shock. To find that your child has just been diagnosed Autistic is a nightmare to most parents. Joining a parent support group may help. Though, in most cases parents need to come to terms with the Autism themselves before they are able to relax and discuss their child with any other person.

The initial shock may shatter all your hopes and aspirations that you may have had for your child. This does not mean that you stop loving your child. The child you have is *your* child and although the diagnosis may have arrived a lot later, you still have to look at your child the same way that you did before the diagnosis. Your Autistic child will reward you in other ways if you help them gain social, communication, physical and academic skills, through your love and support. In my experience the best and most effective way of coping is through love, patience and perseverance.

The initial diagnosis is the time when parents need all the support from family and friends. Many relatives use the words 'he/she will be ok.' This is not offering help rather it is their way of washing their hands of their responsibility. Help is when it is offered genuinely. For example "what can I do to help?"

What to expect of the future
Parents know that they provide the best care for their Autistic child and fear the chances of finding an alternative person to replace that care. At times family members, who are willing or capable to take on the responsibilities of caring for your Autistic child, may not be readily available.

Recognise the strengths and weaknesses in your Autistic child and work on each area of development. The skills could vary from very strong in one area to extremely week in another. The emphasis should be placed mainly on the strengths with a view to help your child move forward and further develop those skills. Obsessions or fixations should be used as motivators towards learning other skills. Steven's interests are animals, music, dance, water, the computer, picture books and DVDs. I focused on these interests to teach him the concept of numbers, activities to develop an understanding of his environment, the meaning of colours, as well as to develop further language.

Most adults with Autism are said to be living at home with their parents or living in a group home. Some high functioning individuals are said to live in supported accommodation with little assistance and a very small proportion are said to be able to live independently. Some have the ability to work but many do not work. Adults with PDD/NOS and Asperger's Syndrome are said to be likely to live independently and likely to be able to work. Although they too experience difficulties in finding work and maintaining a job. The reason for the difficulty in seeking employment is not due to a lack of job skills rather a lack of social skills. Therefore, it is necessary to encourage social skills at an early age to enable them to live and work independently as much as possible.

Predicting your child's potential
Autism is a condition in which we are unable to predict what the future holds for our children. However, it is crucial to focus on priorities. At three, four or five years of age the seriousness of the condition can often be overlooked with the hope that they will cope, achieve or even grow out of it as they get older. While focusing on education and age appropriate skills it is easy to feel

that placing an emphasis on education will benefit your child in the long run. Having given Steven a great deal of educational input myself, I felt let down by the system that I had placed all my faith in. To learn that the schools couldn't show progress leave alone maintain what he had already achieved at home was difficult to comprehend. At times when the progress seemed to be non existent the hopes for his future tended to move further and further away. Receiving less than what Steven needed through the authorities is a result of the struggle that he is currently faced with.

I was caught in a situation where my only option would have been to teach Steven at home myself for a third time on a full time basis. As time went on I put up with whatever Steven received at school. My input was seen as interference at the first school, the second asked for my help in showing them how to teach but did not carry it through with Steven and the third acknowledged my advice but have not shown results of progress in Steven. Having recognised the lack of progress where Steven was showing signs of regression in many areas of his learning, I provided the extra help at home after school. However, my energy level had reached a point where I could only give him so much at the end of a school day. As a result we worked on play activities which he was more willing to participate in. Steven now being a teenager my hopes are that he is taught as many independent and self help skills as possible to one day give him the opportunity to care for himself. The only way to know what to expect of the future is to work on these skills following simple steps that are suited to the child's level and ability. Remember it is important that your child learns to live which means involving the child in helping, coping, fitting in and participating.

Initial concerns
- *Will my child be able to make friends?*
- *Will my child be able to attend a mainstream school?*
- *Will my child be able to care for him/herself?*
- *Will my child ever gain speech?*
- *Will my child be able to walk independently?*
- *Will my child be able to live independently?*
- *Will my child need care for the rest of his/her life?*
- *Will my child be accepted by society?*

Will my child be able to make friends?
Autistic children will play along side other children. Interaction can be taught through turn taking and simple games. Children of family and friends should be encouraged to include Autistic children in social activities to help them first understand the meaning of interaction, join in the interaction and finally enjoy the interaction. Teaching social rules and the meaning of sharing will help in developing friendships.

Will my child be able to attend a mainstream school?
Autistic children vary in their severity and their ability to learn. Some cope very well in mainstream schools with additional support, some do well in special needs schools with or without additional support, some cope well being taught at home and some find it difficult to

cope in any educational setting. What is crucial is to have your child assessed and give your child the level of education that will meet his/her needs.

Will my child be able to care for him/herself?
It is necessary that we deal with the basics when it comes to care while rewarding and encouraging, to further motivate their learning of skills required for everyday living.

Will my child ever gain speech?
A large percentage of children and adults with Autism remain mute. However, until you start working on Speech & Language Therapy it is difficult to assess the level of the impairment. Children with speech disorders need as much Speech & Language Therapy input as possible. Alternatively, teaching sign language together with pictures will offer added support in understanding the meaning of language, whereby minimising the level of frustration caused through a lack of speech.

Will my child be able to walk independently?
The prospect of a child gaining independence through mobility will be of grave concern to parents of children with Autism and associated physical disabilities. However, a child who can be assisted through physiotherapy should be provided the therapy as a matter of priority. In children who have the ability to walk but lack a sense of awareness, an emphasis should be placed on developing coping strategies in dangerous and unsupervised situations. The strategies may involve teaching road safety rules, understanding dangers and following social rules which can be delivered through

table top activities, computer programmes and in the environment in particular. A long and slow process, which will be most effective if the steps followed are simple. For example, teaching the meaning of left and right stop and go, wait and look. These activities are further required to be reinforced using pictures and sequences of events - for example, "what happens if you cross the road when traffic is moving". Prompt answer: "You will get hurt."

Will my child be able to live independently?
It is a hard task to predict the future of our children, but it is possible to work on the areas that need working on. In order to teach the skills associated with independent living the child is required to learn the meaning of the skills being taught. Work towards the long term goal while starting with simple steps.

Will my child need care for the rest of his/her life?
The extent to which an Autistic child will progress is hard to predict. However methods put in place early will offer the child a chance to develop skills required for independent living. The emphasis should be placed on working towards long term goals and thereby, giving your child the best possible chance in life.

Will my child be accepted in society?
There are many ways to teach your child what is socially correct and to be accepted in society. Again this will not happen in an instant, nevertheless it is achievable. The child needs to be included in as many routine and social activities as possible. They could involve a trip to the supermarket, a restaurant, the

cinema or visiting friends. The social interaction is crucial in aiding your child to learn appropriate and acceptable behaviour.

Studying the child's obsessions and using them to create more socially acceptable alternatives that the child takes pleasure in, will help towards social acceptance as well as allow parents and carers to work with the child with more ease. For example, building Lego is more fun than banging on the floor. Hitting a drum is more fun than tapping sticks on the floor. Sitting together doing a puzzle is more fun than picking up bits of soil. All these activities will help create joint attention which will lead to greater social acceptance.

Seeing a happy child is a delightful sight. Autistic children display bizarre behaviour due to being afraid, frustrated, confused or simply as a means of escapism. These are typically expected reactions. Yet, from the position in which the Autistic child stands, the reason for the behaviour manifesting in itself may have to be guessed at. Consequently, the attention needs to be placed on understanding the cause behind the actions to learn how to cope and deal with them, while eventually minimising any negative behaviours. An improper conduct will receive a not so favourable reaction from a society that is less than tolerant of behaviour they do not understand. Therefore, minimising negative behaviour will help towards gaining public acceptance.

Basic skills
- *Toileting care*
- *Washing hands / drying hands*
- *Washing face / drying face*
- *Brushing teeth / rinsing mouth*
- *Washing hair*
- *Washing body*

Areas of basic skills - Not detailed in the book

Eating
- *Use of spoon*
- *Use of fork*
- *Use of knife and fork*
- *Use of knife to cut*
- *Pouring a drink*
- *Opening a packet*

Dressing self
- *Buttoning shirt*
- *Getting clothes on*
- *Getting belt on*
- *Getting socks on*
- *Getting shoes on*
- *Fastening shoes*
- *Tying laces*

TEACHING LIFE SKILLS TO AUTISTIC CHILDREN

Learning to use the toilet
An Autistic child may resist using the toilet when it is a change from what he/she is used to. A reward system will be useful in motivating the child to break the habit. A child, who does not understand the meaning of a reward or lacks the ability to associate the reward with an action, should be rewarded together with the use of an exaggerated amount of praise. A reward can be offered socially, through a favourite food item or a toy. Planning meals at set times each day will help the child fall into a pattern of when it is time to use the toilet. Sitting the child on the toilet immediately after each meal will help encourage motivation through awareness of routine.

Steps to follow:
Sit your child on the toilet. While he/she is seated hold the reward in your hand to remind the child that if the child is successful in using the toilet that this will be the reward. Offer the reward immediately after the child has successfully completed the task so that the child makes a connection between the action and the reward.

How I taught my son
Steven was taught from an early age to enjoy affection. Therefore, when teaching him rejection worked well. Any accidents were dealt by way of asking him to move away from me while refusing any hugs. The praise and the lack of approval was exaggerated to allow Steven to recognise the meaning of his action.

Teaching him the meaning of each facial expression was useful in achieving this task.

Learning to wash his/her hands
Teach your child this task as a lesson activity or a table top activity. This can be achieved through teaching awareness of the hands through imitation.

Steps to follow:
Use child's name-----
Use the prompt: do this------ "Clasp hands"
                              "Rub hands together"
Help a child who has difficulty with imitating an action, by patterning the action for the child using the adult's hands over the child's hands. To assist a child who has no awareness or interest in imitating, the adult requesting the child to imitate the action, should sit facing the child, while the adult patterning the action sits behind the child and helps the child learn the movements of their hands. Once the action has been learnt it should be generalised under running water until the child learns to wash his/her hands independently. At this point the child should also be taught to turn the tap on and off.

Learning to dry his/her hands
Teach your child this task through teaching awareness of fingers and hands through imitation.

Steps to follow:
Use the child's name------
Use the prompt: "do this" ------
"Open hands"

"Close hands"
"Clap hands"
Hold thumb and index finger together
Hold thumb and middle finger together
Hold 2 index fingers together

Once this action has been learnt, generalise the activity using a towel. Pattern the movement of the hands until the task is achieved, whereby the child is able to perform the action independently. To start with, let the child pat dry the hands by leaving the towel on a flat surface. Help the child to pat one side at a time until they are confident of the complete action.

Learning to wash his/her face
Teach your child this action through imitation.
Steps to follow:
Child's name-----
Use the prompt: Do this------ "wash face"
Move your hands over your face using circular motions. Encourage a child who has difficulty in imitating by patterning the child's hands through this activity until he/she is able to perform the action independently. Once the action has been achieved teach the child to cup both hands together by holding hands and pouring water into hands. Use the prompt: "hold water in your hands." Place a basin underneath the child's hands to enable the activity to be performed over and over again without creating much mess. Once both these tasks have been achieved they can be generalised under running water. Pattern the action turn the tap on and turn the tap off. Always use language to support the action in order to encourage learning

through constant association of language and action.

Learning to dry his/her face
Once the child has learnt to dry his/her hands it should be easier to learn to dry the face. If not, this action can be patterned too.

Learning to brush his/her teeth
This is a difficult action for an Autistic child. Therefore, you may be required to pattern the action for a longer period of time than for other actions. The child will need to learn awareness of arm movements, hand movements, wrist movements and the use of facial muscles.

Steps to follow:
Child's name------
Use prompt------ "Brush teeth"
Stand behind the child using your hand over the child's to pattern the action. It will be useful to have a mirror so the child is able to watch the action being patterned. Once the action has been patterned help the child imitate the action again in front of a mirror until he/she has learnt to perform the action independently.

Rinsing mouth
This action should be taught at the same time as brushing teeth.
Steps to follow:
Name of child------
Use prompt: "Rinse mouth"
This action can be taught through imitation.

Washing hair
An action which requires awareness of hands and fingers. Although the movement of the fingers remain consistent the child needs to learn to move the arms at the same time making it a more complex task. The first step can be taught as a lesson activity.

Steps to follow:
Child's name------
Use prompt do this-----"Hold all tips of fingers together and open."
Once the child has learnt this action generalise the skill through patterning the child to wash his/her hair. This action is taught to help the child learn to shampoo his/her own hair. When patterning the action use prompt----- "move your fingers." Once this skill has been achieved the child can be taught to squeeze shampoo into his hands hereby learning to be more independent.

Washing self
Teach the child to imitate this action. The initial step can be done as a lesson activity.

Steps to follow:
Child's name:
Use prompt: do this------ "Move closed hand over body." A mirror will help with imitating the action as it requires awareness of the body together with the coordination of arms, hands and fingers.
Once the action has been learnt, it can be generalised while holding a bar of soap, a sponge or a flannel. At

this point use prompt: ------ "wash with soap."

Brushing hair
An action which will require awareness of arms hand and wrist. It can first be taught as a lesson activity.

Steps to follow:
Child's name--------
Use prompt: do this------ "brush hair"
Pattern the child to move closed hand over his/her head. Once the action has been learnt, teach the child to look at him/herself in the mirror and pattern the action for the child using a hair brush.

TEACHING BODY AWARENESS THROUGH PHYSICAL ACTIVITY

Using a swing
This action requires awareness of arms and legs and will help develop strength in these areas. The swinging motion is an action that most Autistic children enjoy. Therefore, once learnt the child will not need much encouragement to use a swing independently.

Steps to follow:
Childs name:-------
Use prompt------ "Feet up"
"Feet down"
"Pull with your arms"
When teaching an Autistic child to use a swing he/she should be taught to hold on to the swing, while the adult standing in front pushes the swing. This is a good

way to encourage eye contact. Use the prompt: "Feet up" – while the swing is moving forward and use prompt: "feet down" by holding the child's feet and pushing them down allowing the swing to move backwards. Once the child has passed this step and is aware of lifting his/her feet, use the prompt: "can you kick my hands?". The child will pull using his/her arms move body backwards and try to kick your hands. Pattern this action till the child learns the movement and is able to enjoy the activity independently.

Learning to hop
This action will help an Autistic child to learn to balance themselves. When teaching an Autistic child to hop be ready to hold onto him/her to stop them from falling over, which could result in the child resisting the activity. Balancing themselves will be difficult until they learn this action.

Steps to follow:
Child's name------
Use prompt------- stand on one leg. Help the child steady him/herself through the activity and gradually reduce the support to help the child learn to balance independently. Once the child has learnt to balance on one leg use the prompt: jump or hop. I used the prompt jump with Steven as he did not know what hop meant. The next step would be to prompt: jump and move forward while holding the child. Once the action has been achieved, gradually reduce support in order to encourage independent hopping. Steven was just becoming aware of the hopping movement, when I called a few children in the playground and asked them

if they could show Steven how to hop. It was great fun as most of the children in the playground joined where we all hopped together and the skill was learnt in no time.

Learning to throw / catch a ball

This activity will require 2 people to assist the child. One to pattern the throwing and catching action, and the other to throw the ball to the child.

Steps to follow:
Child's name-----
Use prompt-------"Throw ball"
             "Catch ball"

The person patterning the child will hold the ball using the child's hands while easing the child's hands off the ball to perform the throwing action. To catch the ball the person throwing should throw the ball straight to the child's hands while the person patterning should help the child cup the hands and keep them cupped to receive the ball. Once the child starts to become aware of the action reduce the patterning while encouraging the child to perform the action independently. During this activity, encourage the child to look at the ball, anticipate and wait for the ball and catch the ball.

Learning to kick a ball

Place the ball by the child's feet and kick the ball.
If the child is not paying attention repeat the action. If the child has no awareness of the kicking movement pattern the action for the child.

Steps to follow:
Child's name----
Use prompt------ kick ball.
Hold the child's foot from behind move the foot forward to perform the kicking action. Once the child is able to perform this action stand a few feet away from the child and kick the ball back to the child. Gradually increase the distance to encourage a harder kick through awareness of strength in legs and feet. This is a good way to encourage social interaction through meaningful play.

Learning to bounce a ball
Use a large ball to perform this action. Teach the child to bounce a ball using your hand over child's hand.

Steps to follow:
Child's name-----
Use prompt------ bounce ball
Once the child is aware of the bouncing movement alternate the action with the child. Once the action has been learnt encourage the child to perform the action independently.

Learning to enjoy a roundabout / scooter
An action which requires awareness of the complete body. The child will need to learn to push the roundabout using arms and move the revolving platform with the feet while placing one foot on the ground and the other on the platform.
This action needs awareness of language and awareness of imitation.

Steps to follow:
Child's name------
Use prompt------"Push with your arms"
"One foot on platform one foot down."
" Keep moving"
Perform the action in the same way that the child needs to learn the action. Push the roundabout while moving in front of the child so the child can learn to imitate the action. Once the child has learnt this action he/she will also be able to use a scooter.

Learning to ride a tricycle / bike
An action which requires awareness of the complete body. The child is required to recognise direction in moving the handle bars as well as the pedals.

Steps to follow:
Child's name------
Use prompt-------"Ride bike"
"Move forward"
"Move backwards"
"Turn left / Turn right"
"Turn around"
"Stop"
"Wait"
Perform the action for the child while the child is sat on the seat of the tricycle turning the handle bars and the pedals at the same time. Ensure you keep your hands safe from getting trapped while moving the pedals. Stop the action while pushing for a while and use the prompt: "move forward" to allow the child to use his/her awareness of the how the tricycle moves. Continue to do so until the child is motivated enough to

enjoy the activity without the support. Steven was a child who completely resisted the activity while screaming all the way while attempting to get off his tricycle. I somehow persevered through a battle of wills, as I knew he would enjoy it once he learnt the activity. Once he learnt the activity he not only learnt to enjoy it but he was on the tricycle at all times, while at times he peddled to watch TV.

CHAPTER NINE

DEALING WITH THE PUZZLE IN THE BRAIN

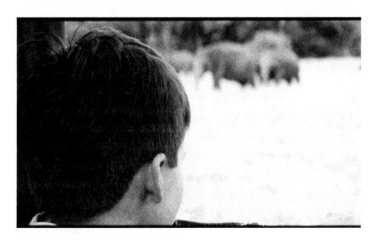

My first thought of teaching Steven was to find the best way of getting through to him. Nor was the Autism alone a puzzle the world itself seemed a puzzle to him. Watching Steven very closely and testing his knowledge helped me in learning to see the world through his eyes. In an effort to help him I had to review the complexities of the world and find ways of inputting all this information into his Autistic brain. Since Steven was good at jigsaw puzzles, I looked at the world as a series of jigsaw puzzles and thought of as many ways as possible to put these puzzles together. Having observed Steven I recognised his interests as elephants, horses, music, water, dance, Disney DVDs, the computer and other animals. Steven enjoyed an elephant safari in Sri Lanka as well as four days in Disney land, Paris. These interests were developed in

Steven at two years of age. His interest in water meant he was ready to strip off to get into a pond, a lake, the sea, a swimming pool or even a fountain. He had to be taught when and where it was acceptable to get into the water.

Most people cannot comprehend what it is like for an Autistic child to fit into our world. Having tried very hard to put myself into my son's brain and his way of thinking, I not only learnt to empathise but felt the strength in him. I gained the strength and motivation through my admiration for Steven who lacked all the tools that we all take so much for granted, when learning to deal with our world. It all comes so naturally to us all where as every step towards living in our world is a great effort in terms of learning as well as coping for Steven. Have strength in your self and learn to accept your strength and responsibility and this will be the brightest start of your child's future. Learn the meaning of trust and simplicity. I never expected to be able to develop the patience and skills to teach an Autistic child. I found it challenging though extremely rewarding.

Teaching Steven awareness of himself

I first looked at what was most important in the learning process and decided it was to teach awareness of himself and his immediate world. I chose the face as the first topic. I took two photographs of Steven's face and enlarged them to life size to help him recognise his own face easily. I cut out the eyes, the ears, the nose and the mouth and laminated the individual parts as well as the complete face. The individual parts had

Velcro backing and the complete face had Velcro stuck on the position where each individual shape had to be positioned.

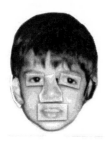 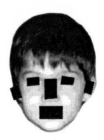

Teaching Steven to recognise his senses

To start teaching I sat Steven at the table facing me and held the picture of his face and pointed to each individual part of the face on the picture. I named each part eyes, nose, mouth and ears giving time for Steven to touch his own or move his hand to each part. At times when he didn't respond I guided his hand through each step.

In realising that Steven experienced difficulty in recognising himself, I sat him in front of a full length mirror and worked on recognition of his own face by asking him to touch his face. It was interesting to note that he would continuously look back to check if there was anyone else standing or sitting behind him while touching the mirror to check if he could reach the other child.

Once Steven was able to identify parts of his face in himself I gave him the Velcro shape of each part of the face to position correctly on the shape of the face that was on the laminated card. The next step was to teach Steven awareness of his senses. During this stage of learning it was necessary to use rewards that would motivate Steven. I wasn't too keen on the idea of food rewards and used a box of favourite toys instead.

I held the picture of the eyes and asked the question "what do you see with?" I gave Steven time to touch his eyes and prompted the response "I see with my eyes". Once Steven learnt awareness of his eyes I helped him generalise the skill. I did this by holding a single object at a time at Steven's eye level while asking the question "what do you see". For this task I used the most obvious objects that Steven came into contact with during his day together with favourite toys - for example, cup, plate, spoon, fork, knife, video, horse, and elephant.

Once Steven learnt to associate his eyes with seeing I further generalised the skill by introducing pictures of every day objects, activities, situations and places by asking the question what do you see while prompting the response. I allowed Steven enough time to think and recall the word that he was looking for before prompting the word. This was done to stop Steven becoming too dependent on the prompt while offering him encouragement to learn with the minimum level of frustration.

Once Steven learnt awareness of his eyes the next step was to teach awareness of his ears. This was done through using different sounds. I used a sound track cassette for this task as well as a home recording of everyday sounds. I held the pictures of the ears in front of Steven and asked the question "what do you hear with?" I prompted the response "I hear with my ears".

The sound track lotto consisted of four cards indicating nine pictures on each card together with counters to place on each picture once the sound had been heard and recognised. I colour copied and laminated the sound track cards and cut them out to help Steven identify the sounds individually, prior to using the card that showed all nine pictures. The reason for cutting the pictures out individually was to mix the placement of the cards to help learn that Steven understood the sounds rather than following a pattern with the sounds he had heard. (Rote learning rather than thinking and understanding). I organised the laminated cards in a pack and numbered them at the back of each card, so that they would correspond with the sound heard on the soundtrack tape.

To start with I held the pictures up in front of Steven one at a time to introduce him to the sounds that he was to hear. For example, I held the picture of the dog in front of Steven and prompted "Dog". I did the same with all the pictures until I was sure that Steven was able to identify each sound with the corresponding picture.

Prior to starting I used the command "Steven it is time

to listen" "I listen with my ears". I placed the first 3 laminated sound pictures on the table and played the sound track. I gave Steven a counter and asked Steven the question "what do you hear"? When he placed the counter on the correct picture I said "I hear ------". I repeated the same steps for all the sounds using three pictures at a time. When he was able to sustain his attention to identify the sounds in more than three pictures, I increased the number to six pictures followed by nine and finally to all thirty six pictures. Steven enjoyed this activity and was easily motivated whereby he learnt fast and well.

Once Steven was able to place the counters on all the pictures without any prompt I worked on his listening without the pictures. I used the command "Steven it is time to listen" and "what do you hear?". When teaching Steven "a" and "the" were deliberately left out to prevent any confusion in associating "the" and "a" as part of the word.

We worked on as many sounds as possible. At this stage Steven didn't need any prompting to recall the word for the sound he had heard.

Steven learnt to respond appropriately to all the sounds introduced to him. Steven was encouraged to listen through first introducing him to sounds of Animals which have always been his favourite interest.

Teaching Steven to recognise environmental sounds

I hear dog	I hear thunder	I hear sea	I hear drinking
I hear cow	I hear fire works	I hear aero plane	I hear flute
I hear bird	I hear owl	I hear car	I hear rain
I hear elephant	I hear frog	I hear fire engine	I hear piano
I hear duck	I hear cat	I hear tractor	I hear drums
I hear horse	I hear sheep	I hear motorbike	I hear sneezing
I hear pig	I hear baby crying	I hear digging sand	I hear cutting paper
I hear hen	I hear ball bouncing	I hear splashing water	I hear door shutting
I hear coughing	I hear running water	I hear pouring water	I hear eating crisps

Once Steven learnt awareness of his ears the next step was to teach him the functions of his mouth. For this activity I asked the question "what do you talk with?" and prompted Steven with the response, "I talk with my mouth" and "I eat with my mouth". For this activity I placed play food items on the table and introduced Steven to each food item separately. I held each play food item in front of Steven and prompted the response for each item. I introduced Steven to as many food items as possible. Once Steven had learnt to identify food and non food, to further explain the concept, I placed three items on the table 2 non food items and one food item. I asked the question, "Steven, what do you eat?" I helped guide Steven's hand to the food item and prompted the response "I eat------------"

Teaching Steven to associate food with eating

I eat sausages	I eat grapes	I eat pear	I eat carrot
I eat bread	I eat strawberry	I eat sweets	I eat apple
I eat pizza	I eat yoghurt	I eat marshmallow	I eat snack bar
I eat spaghetti	I eat ice cream	I eat jelly babies	I eat chicken
I eat fish fingers	I eat mango	I eat rice	I eat potato
I eat porridge	I eat Weetabix	I eat Corn flakes	I eat egg

Once Steven was able to identify the functions of his mouth the next step was to teach him awareness of his nose. I held the picture of his nose and asked the question "what do you smell with?" I prompted the response "I smell with my nose". I placed a flower and a bar of soap in front of Steven and held each one to my nose and sniffed to help Steven imitate the action. He found it difficult at first but once we sat in front of the mirror he was able to imitate after a few attempts and understood the function of his nose. I gave the soap to Steven's hand and asked the question "what do you smell" and prompted the answer "I smell soap" and did the same with flower.

Once Steven was able to understand and identify the use of his senses. I asked him five questions which he learnt understood and responded to without a prompt.

Teaching Steven the functions of his senses

"What do you see with?"	"I see with my eyes"
"What do you hear with?"	"I hear with my ears"
"What do you eat with?"	"I eat with my mouth"
"What do you smell with?"	"I smell with my nose"
"What do you touch with?"	"I touch with my hand"

We next moved onto body parts. For this activity I found a very useful puzzle of a boy, which had the boy's body as a picture in the centre of the puzzle. I laid out the three part puzzle of the boy separately and the body parts separately. The individual parts of the body surrounded the main puzzle.

I picked up each part of the puzzle starting with the head and asked Steven to identify each part on him self - for example, "Touch Steven's head".

We worked through to identify as many parts of the body starting with parts of the head. It was necessary that Steven learnt to relate to his body in order to teach him to use his body to participate in play or self help activities. To help Steven through this activity I held the picture in front of him and helped him move his hand to identify the part on his body.

Teaching Steven to identify parts of his body

Touch Steven's head	Touch Steven's feet
Touch Steven's face	Touch Steven's toes
Touch Stevens's eyes	Touch Steven's back
Touch Stevens's ears	Touch Steven's hair
Touch Steven's nose	Touch Steven's legs
Touch Steven's mouth	Touch Steven's stomach
Touch Steven's chin	Touch Steven's shoulders
Touch Steven's cheeks	Touch Steven's knees
Touch Steven's neck	Touch Steven's elbows
Touch Steven's arms	Touch Steven's hands
Touch Steven's bottom	Touch Steven's fingers

Once Steven learnt to associate with parts of his body he was more able to learn activities through imitation. Since most actions used in every day activities seem complex for an individual who does not understand the meaning of imitation, it was necessary to break down the activities to simple movements. All physical activities fit into two categories which involve gross and fine motor movement. The use of limbs and body movements being gross motor and the use of hands together with fingers being fine motor.

I started by teaching Steven gross motor skills. This was done by sitting or standing facing Steven and doing an action while giving the command Steven do this------. I called out the action so that he could associate the language with the action.

I gave a moment for Steven to imitate the action and at times when he wasn't able to follow the action, I helped guide his hands to achieve the action. He was helped through the movements until he was able to perform them independently.

Teaching imitation of gross motor movements

Put your arms up	Tap table
Put your arms out	Clap hands
Wave your arms	Shake your head
Circle your arms	Nod your head
Bend your arms	Turn around
Stamp your feet	Cover your face with hands
Jump	Tap shoulders
March	Stand on one leg
Knock	Move body from side to side
Put your hands on your waist	Tap your head

The next step was to teach Steven awareness of his hands. I started by sitting facing Steven. I gave the command 'do this' as in gross motor imitation. At times when he indicated difficulty with imitating I placed my hand over his and helped him through the action. I gradually reduced the guidance to enable him to perform the action independently.

Teaching imitation of fine motor movements

Clap hands	Wiggle fingers
Clasp hands	Touch thumb and index finger
Make a fist	Touch thumbs
Thumbs up	Rub hands together
Thumbs down	Bend fingers one at a time
Give me five	Tap fingers on the table

Once Steven learnt to imitate gross and fine motor movements we worked on activities to further develop these skills.

Teaching Steven to use a pencil

For this activity it is possible to either use a tripod grip or work without. I found the two together was the most effective for Steven. This way he didn't get too dependent on the tripod grip. In order to start this activity I sat Steven at a low table and sat beside him to be able to best support him through the activity.

Since this was the first step towards writing I gave Steven a sheet of paper and let him scribble as freely as he wanted. I used the command: "Steven draw" and gave him time to become familiar with the pencil. Following the awareness of pencil on paper, I used a few basic stencil shapes starting with a triangle, square and circle moving onto more detailed shapes. In addition I created my own dot to dot sheets which helped Steven develop and maintain his attention.

While Steven was sat at the table using the pencil, I

helped him by placing my hand over his. To assist him with the proper pencil grip, I guided his hand to hold the pencil using the thumb, the index finger and the middle finger and added pressure on the other two fingers so that he learnt to keep them bent while using the pencil. Once he had a feel for the pencil grip we worked on activities to help towards writing and drawing.

I used many dot to dot activities to encourage moving the pencil from one point to the other as well as tracing activities. Steven learnt to trace very simple shapes to more detailed shapes. As Steven showed an interest in tracing I kept the shapes inconsistent to help further develop his attention.

Once Steven showed some awareness of the use of his hands to perform writing activities I created additional work sheets to help towards independent drawing. I took a blank A4 sheet of paper and drew a vertical line on the centre of the page and divided it to four horizontal lines. The purpose of this was to allow me to draw in the box on the left and to teach Steven to copy the same in the box on the right.

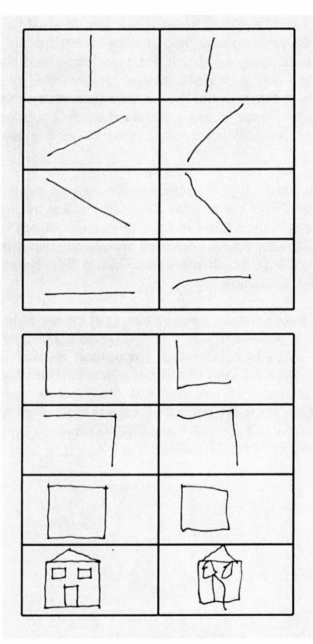

238

I drew a vertical line in the first box on the left and used the command: "Steven do same" – "draw line." I gave the pencil to Steven to copy the same line in the box next to it on the right. I guided Steven's hand over his pencil grip to draw the line. I continued to support and gradually reduced the support to allow Steven to draw a line independently. The same process was followed for the next three boxes by drawing two diagonal lines in opposite directions and one horizontal line. This is the first step towards learning to draw using straight lines. I used the prompts, "line across" to draw a horizontal line and "line down" to draw a vertical line. In addition I used the prompts "draw diagonal line," "draw square" and "draw house."

Teaching Steven to colour within a shape

For this activity I created the first work sheet comprising of the basic shapes: circle, square, triangle, rectangle, heart, diamond and star. The activity had to be made easy to motivate Steven to colour. Therefore, we used easy to apply smooth wax crayons or felt tips. However, wax crayons seemed to work better in developing his concentration. Pencil crayons seemed to need more pencil pressure and effort and were to be worked on later once the motivation had developed.

I gave the wax crayon to Steven's hand, called out the colour and used the command, for example, Steven colour the circle blue. While he coloured I guided his hand to ensure that he stayed within the lines. Prompting: "colour inside circle". At this point since the emphasis was on colouring rather than learn colours we focused on the single activity of colouring by only using the name of the colour and the shape once or twice during the activity.

Once Steven had learnt colours and shapes during separate activities he was able to associate colour and shape and colour in the appropriate shape using the crayon he was requested to use.

Learning to associate colours with objects or what he sees in his environment meant we were able to further develop an understanding in this area by using individual colouring sheets for each colour.

I created a work sheet for the red colouring using drawings of a strawberry, an apple, a rose and a heart. A sheet for the yellow colouring using drawings of a banana, a lemon, the sun and the moon. A sheet for the green colouring using drawings of a frog, a turtle, a leaf, a snake and grass. A sheet for the blue colouring using drawings of blueberries, a bird and a hat. A sheet for the orange colouring using drawings of a monkey, an orange and a shirt. A sheet for the white colouring using drawings of a cloud, a sheet of paper and a rabbit. A sheet for the black colouring using drawings of a dog, the road and shoes. A sheet for the purple colouring using drawings of grapes, a crayon, and a coat. A sheet for the pink colouring using drawings of a pig, a flower and a button. A sheet for the brown colouring using drawings of a horse, a cow and a dog. A sheet for the grey colouring using drawings of an elephant, a rabbit and trousers.

Teaching Steven the meaning of colours
To teach Steven the concept of colours we worked with a variety of different materials. We used coloured reels, colour matching cards, play dough together with coloured pictures and photographs.

We started by matching pictures using four picture cards which consisted of six pictures on each. I laid two cards on the table at a time. The cards represented one colour on each card. Steven being visually strong was able to match the blue pictures to the blue card, the yellow pictures to the yellow card, the green pictures to the green card, and the red pictures to the red card quite easily.

For the next activity, I cut out 10cm squares in each colour and laminated them. I first laid the red and blue cards on the table in front of Steven and held a red reel up and asked Steven to "give me red". As Steven was good at colour matching he didn't need to be prompted to give me the correct colour. We followed the same rule for all the colours laying the cards out starting with two at a time and increasing them to more cards as he further developed his attention.

Once Steven started to become familiar with colours, I laid the cards out again two at a time. I gave my hand out and used the command: "Steven give me ---for example, red. I gave him time to look at both colours watching his eyes all along. At times when he hadn't paid attention to the command, I repeated the prompt while circling my index finger around the cards to direct his attention. I repeated the word "red" and if I still didn't receive a correct response I guided Steven's hand to the red card and helped him pick it up by placing my hand over his and prompted him to give it to my hand by holding my hand out. I recognised at this point that although Steven was able to match colours very easily that he had a great deal of difficulty in remembering and recalling the "word associated with the command". This meant that he had a poor auditory memory which was causing a barrier towards his learning. He required repetition and patience to help develop that memory.

Once Steven learnt one colour I took the learnt colour away and placed another card whereby always showing two cards on the table. I shuffled the cards quickly around the table to different positions to encourage Steven to look. Steven was expected to listen to the command, process the command, look at the two cards, make the selection and give it to my hand. For many normally developing children actions involving selections comes automatically, but Steven needed to be taught each step separately.

To teach colours expressively the most effective method was to use the environment and objects associated with everyday living. This process taught Steven to recognise learning different shades of the same colour as well as to learn that certain colours could remain constant. I used the same colour cards as well as pictures and objects. I held up a colour card and asked the question: What colour is it? Or held an object and asked what colour is, for example, ball? The awareness of colours was further generalised by associating it with shapes.

I cut out and laminated the most standard shapes in as many colours and worked with Steven to develop his receptive language by using the command: "Steven give me Yellow circle". Once he was able to associate colour with the shape I held up a shape and asked the question...e.g.: "what colour is the triangle?".

Teaching Steven to use scissors
The function of cutting using a pair of scissors, teaches a variety of fine motor co-ordination skills. To start with it was necessary to use hand over hand guidance.

I found that an A4 sheet of paper would be awkward for Steven to hold onto while cutting as it tended to flop easily and could be more of a distracter towards learning the skill. Therefore, I decided to fold the A4 sheet in half along the width of the paper and tear it into two equal parts. I used this size for all the cutting activities. I didn't choose card as it is more difficult to cut using scissors which would have reduced his level of motivation.

The first exercise was to cut along a straight line. I drew a horizontal line along the width of the paper and helped Steven hold the paper with his left hand using his thumb and index finger while placing my hand over his. Steven being a right hander, we used this hand to manipulate the scissors. I used a safe pair of children's scissors and helped Steven to place his thumb through one gripping section of the scissors and place his index and middle finger through the other. The grip section of the scissors needed to have adequate space for my fingers to go through them in order to support Steven's grip.

We cut along the line very slowly. I used the command "Steven cut paper" while supporting Stevens's right hand to cut the paper and his left hand to hold and guide the paper. Since this was the start of the cutting activity Steven kept losing his concentration and let me do the cutting but as time went on he got a feel for the use of the scissors and the cutting activity. I gradually reduced the hand on hand cutting in a way that when he finally learnt to cut he didn't realize that he was cutting on his own.

Once Steven was able to cut along the line without support as well as hold the paper we moved onto cutting shapes. I drew the shapes as large as possible on the half A4 sheet and started from the simplest shape and moved onto more detailed shapes.

1	"L"	6	"Triangle"	11	"Diamond"	16	"Flower"
2	"Arc"	7	"Rectangle"	12	"Star"	17	"Tree"
3	"C"	8	"Circle"	13	"Boat"	18	"Lamp"
4	"V"	9	"Oval"	14	"Car"	19	"Vase"
5	"Square"	10	"Heart"	15	"House"	20	"Duck"

CHAPTER TEN

RESEARCH ON AUTISM

Research is carried out on genetic, biochemical, physiological and psychological forms of the disorder. In order to gain a more complete understanding of Autism, scientists are using new imagery techniques showing the living brain in more detailed action. This method has allowed closer observation with greater clarity. The clarity indicates how the brain changes when an individual is performing mental tasks, makes movements or speaks. Hereby, allowing scientists to locate the areas in the brain which are associated with those actions. Furthermore, Autism has been described as 'autoimmune system disorder' as it has been discovered that the Autistic child's immune system is compromised genetically and or environmentally.

It has been noted that around 75% of individuals with Autism accompany learning disabilities where 15%-30% of them experience seizures. In addition Autism affects around five in ten thousand with a male to female ratio of 4:1. Some have shown a great deal of talent indicating exceptional skills in drawing, mathematics or in the field of music. Autistic spectrum disorders are said to affect the lives of over 500.000 families in the UK with girls showing more severe symptoms and greater cognitive impairment.

Cause: No single identifiable cause. Genetic factors, genetically mediated vulnerabilities to the environment and chemical abnormalities in the brain which fail to produce enzymes are all said to be causes. Furthermore, problems during pregnancy, delivery, birth, environmental factors (possible toxins from the environment) and viral infections have been said to trigger Autism in a person who is genetically susceptible.

In addition, Autism is more common in individuals who display medical conditions such as Fragile X Syndrome, Tuberous Sclerosis and Congenital Rubella Syndrome, while harmful substances in the system during pregnancy have also been associated with Autism.

Researchers are investigating the chances of a cluster of unstable genes which could interfere with the development of the brain. Tests have been carried out on chromosome sites that have been found to be significant particularly on chromosome 7 and 15. It is said to be likely that the incidence of Autism results from the interaction of a small number of specific genes and possibly with some external factor. However, these genes have not yet been pinned down but may include HOXA1 gene, which is active in the brain stem at the time of development, when the first neurons are forming in the embryo. Furthermore, researchers have located seven genes prevalent among individuals with Autism. Some speculate that Autism is not a single condition but a group of several conditions that manifest in similar ways. Scientists have used a technique called gene splicing which enables them to manipulate microscopic bits of gene and find abnormal genes that could be a factor in Autism. Furthermore, research is being carried out to find a link between Autism and other brain disorders.

Scientists with NIMH (National Institute of Mental Health) state that as the data on brain chemicals is accumulated they are closer to developing or reversing imbalances and hope that one day the ability may be there to prevent the disorder or when scientists learn more about genetic transmission of Autism they may be able to replace the defective gene even before the infant is born.

What ever the cause, it seems clear that babies with Autism are either born with it or have it in their system and develop it later. Bad parenting or psychological factors in a child's development is not known to cause Autism.

Carnagie Mellon's Centre for cognitive brain imaging have discovered through scans carried out on the brains of high functioning Autistic individuals that certain regions of the brain do not communicate with each other as in the brains of non Autistic individuals. They conclude that this break down explains why people with Autism lack common sense, recognition of faces, and the ability to understand emotions. The synchronisation is said to be particularly poor in the language processing areas.

Increase in the prevalence of Autism

To determine how many people have Autism has been difficult as there is no central register of everyone who has Autism. However, the results of surveys since 50 years ago when it was first recognised by Leo Kanner has lead to an increase in awareness indicating an increase in the prevalence of Autism. Recent studies have estimated 1 in 100 children with Autistic Spectrum Disorders while a rough estimate of the UK population has been estimated at over 500,000 affected with ASD.

Medication
Scientists have found no medication to rectify the brain structures or impaired nerve connections related to Autism. Drugs to treat similar symptoms related to behaviour are said to aid people with Autism. Medications used for anxiety and depression have relieved some symptoms though they may not work for every individual with Autism. NIMH research found that clomipramine a medication used for treating obsessive compulsive behaviour worked to minimise obsessive and repetitive behaviour.

Vitamin B6 together with magnesium stimulates brain function. The reason being that vitamin B6 helps create enzymes that are required in the brain, while magnesium is an essential mineral which is necessary for the healthy function of all cells in the body and the brain. Although magnesium deficiency is said to be rare, children with Autism have shown inadequate levels of the mineral.

Side effects
Drugs could have side effects and should only be administered by a doctor.

Hyperactivity
A behaviour which is associated with ADHD (Attention Deficit and Hyperactive Disorder). Hyperactivity which is sometimes associated with Autism has shown that the stimulant Ritalin has been used in treating ADHD symptoms. In addition research indicates that drugs have been most effective when given to higher functioning children without any signs of seizures or any other neurological disorder.

Having read up on Ritalin as well as discussed its side effects with a developmental paediatrician I was not prepared to try the drug for Steven. However, the staff at the second primary school that Steven attended in the UK spoke of its benefits and urged me to put him on the drug. With a great deal of reluctance, I agreed to start him on it with the smallest possible dose. The staff at the school were pleased as he was quiet and manageable, though they weren't able to show any progress in his learning. Furthermore, once he returned home from school when the drug had worn off, he indicated distress combined with hyperactive behaviour, aggression, an erratic sleep pattern and loss of appetite. Steven had been on Ritalin for a month and I wasn't happy with what it was doing to his system. I stopped the drug despite the school's efforts to try and get him back on it, as I felt he didn't need it. I recognised that he was far happier and more focused without it. Although the drug calmed him during the day its effects resulted in negative behaviour once the drug had worn off. I wasn't prepared to get him dependent on a drug which was damaging to his health. I opted to work on his diet and exercise which was far more effective in managing his behaviour.

Some scientists believe that some children in families are more likely to be Autistic due to similarities in disorders running in the family. The exact cause for Autism has been extremely difficult to diagnose due to the complexities of the human brain.

The human brain which consists of over a hundred billion nerve cells called neurons, connect with hundreds of thousands of other cells in the brain and body to help us function. The neurons help the functions of our senses work together.

Scientists are in the process of looking at areas where the connections in the brain of an Autistic individual are affected. They have indicated damage or lacking in development in the areas of communication and emotion, while showing a neurologically immature hippocampus. The hippocampus which is the key factor in sensory input, learning and memory where information is sent from the senses to the hippocampus which processors what is received and transfers it onto the cerebral cortex for long term storage. It has been said that the message which is not transferred effectively from the hippocampus is a result of auditory processing problems in Autistic children.

Social behaviour
A dysfunction in social behaviour is the key defining feature of Autism. A theory said that Autistic individuals do not receive 'biochemical' pleasure from being with people. Beta-endorphins is a substance

released in the brain during social behaviour. Autistic individuals are said to show high levels of beta-endorphin suggesting that the Autistic individual is not dependant on social interaction to gain pleasure. Furthermore, research has shown that the drug Naltrexone which blocks the performance of beta-endorphins has indicated increased social behaviour.

It is said that the Autistic individual's brain has been found to have an underdeveloped amygdala and hippocampus which are both parts of the limbic system. The amygdala is responsible for emotional function, aggression and sensory processing while the hippocampus is responsible for the function of learning, memory and integrating the sensors.

In addition individuals with high functioning Autism or Aspergers Syndrome are said to have immaturities in the amygdala though only slight or no impairments in the hippocampus indicating the reason as to why these individuals intellectual doesn't correspond with their emotional development.

Theories of Autism
Evidence through brain research supports dysfunctions in Autism to four areas of the brain. These involve the amygdala, the Frontal Lobes, the Temporal Lobe and the Cerebellum. The amygdala which lies in the Temporal Lobe receives sensory input from other brain structures. Amygdala damage is said to be the cause for individuals with Autism being unable to connect their mother's face with comfort or develop early social bonds which are seen necessary in normal

development. In addition the amygdala is said to respond to ambiguous situations in the environment that protect us by sending a warning signal to increase our sense of awareness. Damage to the amygdala suggests the result of high levels of anxiety in Autistic individuals.

Research suggests that the human mind and nervous system remain plastic for a longer period than previously believed and that individuals with Autism have been known to develop cognitively throughout their lives.

Scientists have said that the evidence that they have found indicates multiple deficits in the structure and function of the brain, to be the cause of Autism. Therefore, it has been acknowledged that it is extremely difficult to point to one area of the brain to suggest the damage to that particular area as being the cause for Autism.

Genetics of Autism
There has been constant disagreement over the vulnerability of genes to environmental triggers or the role of genes in the etiology of Autism. Researchers have been viewing genetics as the underlying cause. However, it has made research more indistinguishable as most Autistic children were seen to have apparently neuro-typical parents. This finding has suggested that Autism is not the cause of a single gene rather a cluster of genes.

Researchers who have been searching for the root

causes for Autism over the past twenty years have recently come close to discovering a handful of genes and chromosomes that could be responsible for the various aspects of the disorder.

The discovery of such genes have proved difficult due to the complex nature of Autism and the variability in symptoms together with abilities, and the degree in which the individuals are affected. Researchers have said that Autism could be linked to the possibility of two or more of a large number of genes explaining that a person with Autism could have mutations in several genes.

The most promising find reported is that the gene connected to Autism may be on the long arm of chromosome 15. Near the Centro mere which is said to be the indented part which holds the two sides of the chromosome together. The region has been said to be well known for genetic abnormalities such as duplication of the chromosome DNA. Although short duplication does not cause any apparent harm longer duplications are said to carry a 50% chance of developing Autism.

British scientists are said to have identified a group of genes that are responsible for the cause of Autism, reaching closer and closer to a cure and treatment for the most complex and least understood of mental disorders. Using these findings the scientists will be analysing the genes in order to determine effective treatments towards helping Autistic people in the future. The nature of the gene is said to provide future medical help for Autism.

Children with gene variant are said to have double the risk of developing the disorder. In addition Autism is said to be linked to the MET Gene as well as other environmental factors. The MET gene which is active before birth and after birth is responsible for the development of the cerebral cortex and helps build the cerebellum, both areas which are defective have resulted in inactivity in these areas in Autistic individuals.

Research suggests that some parts of Autistic adult's brains do not seem to communicate with other areas of the brain, calling it the "disconnect hypothesis" where it is said that the structure of the circuits may be different.

Abnormal levels of serotonin have been found in the brains of Autistic children which is said to be a possibility in the problems associated with regulation of mood.

Scientists have found that relatives of individuals could show signs of Autistic brain differences without being Autistic. A finding which is said to make it easier to pin point families likely to be at risk of having a child with Autism.

Comparing brain scans of parents of Autistic children against brain scans of parents of non Autistic children indicated that the brains of parents of Autistic children shared similar structural differences to that of their child as well as showed an increase in the motor cortex and the basal ganglia which is the area related to movement, planning and imitation. It was also said to be evident that the somatosensory cortex the area which is responsible for reading social information was smaller than average.

Research indicated that the brain messenger acetylcholine in Autistic individuals indicate less receptors while showing more cramped in columns of neurons in the Cerebral Cortex. Furthermore, it has been recognised that children with Autism were less able to differentiate between sounds that were similar.

Scientists have found a gene linked to Autism and believe that a risk assessment test will be on the market in the near future. The gene has been found in chromosome sixteen and is said to be evident that the EN2 gene is an Autism gene. However, contrary to the studies recent research suggests that there is no link between the two.

The Cerebellum and Autism
The Cerebellum which is located near the brain stem is responsible for motor movements. Damage caused to this area results in Cerebral Palsy leaving an individual affected by this disorder to lose control of their motor movements. Recent research indicates that the Cerebellum is also responsible for the development of speech and attention, recognition of emotion and the ability to learn.

Dr. Eric Courchesne through examining structural brain

abnormalities in Autistic individuals found that two areas of the Cerebellum, Lobules VI and VII were a great deal smaller in Autistic individuals. This abnormality is referred to as 'hyperplasia'. Having researched the two Lobules Dr. Courchesne has discovered a relationship connected to the lobules, between shifting attention in a timely manner which is a primary difficulty in Autism. The time taken in shifting attention means that, they lose the context and content of what has been said.

Structural differences in the Autistic brain

Autism becomes apparent in early childhood and is the most severe of pervasive developmental disorders. Autistic individuals behave in a way that is not normal to that of a neuro typical individual. Scientists while assuming that the behaviours originate from the brain have made comparisons in the structural differences of the Autistic and the neuro typical brain. The size of the different parts of the brain is said to be disproportionate or distorted in the Autistic brain. All aspects of Autism is said to be caused by the decreased connectivity within the Corpus Callosum resulting in the brain's internal communication to diminish. Many scientists have acknowledged the idea that Autism manifests in many regions of the brain.

Motivation to talk

In most typical situations motivation to talk comes from a desire to share thoughts, interest in other people as well as gaining attention. The self directed interests of an Autistic individual means that, a motivation to talk needs to be developed through the interests that they possess within themselves. A non verbal Autistic child may reach for something they want accompanied by some form of vocalisation, instead of pointing and using eye contact as an effective means of communication. Researchers assumed in the past that the spoken language in an individual, developed through the pre wiring where every human being was born with an inbuilt ability to talk. Today researchers believe that the social and emotional aspects of language are an equally important factor to linking words together to stringing a sentence. The ability to detect emotion in tone and recognise the sound level in the voice are of significance in reading and understanding a message that is delivered verbally.

Researchers found a new phenomenon to explain the brain cells called mirror neurons which are responsible for the act of imitation in babies. Baby's brains are programmed to imitate and reflect emotions and actions. An indication, that observing another person in pain will trigger the same cells that react to our own pain.

The mind blindness of an Autistic individual explains the inability to interact with or understand the thoughts of others. Researchers have said that individuals with Autism have faulty mirror neurons which results in an inability to imitate. The inability to read others makes it difficult for the Autistic individual to develop meaningful language, while an ability to use language with an awareness of its impact on another's mind has been constantly used to manipulate others. This lack of awareness gives the Autistic individual an added disadvantage when learning to live in a complex and confusing world. Messages conveyed through eye contact or body language would be completely lost on an Autistic individual.

Autistic individuals vary in their impairment showing variability in symptoms and levels of functioning. Some indicate normal levels of intelligence and develop language skills, while others develop very little or no language, while a child who is mildly affected by Autism may result in a late diagnosis of the condition which could lead to a lack of support from an early age.

Brain imaging
NIMH scientists are carrying out studies which involve brain imaging, tissue banks, animal models, genetics, development neurobiology and neuropsychological aspects of disorders. Their aim is to spread awareness, form an accurate diagnosis and find effective methods of treatment.

MRI scans offer a great deal of potential towards learning and understanding the emotional and intellectual deficits of Autism and other neuropsychiatry disorders. However, the limitation in the amount of data that scientists have accumulated on the function of the normal brain and it's development makes it difficult to compare the differences with that of the Autistic brain. As a result of the lack of data the NIMH is co-sponsoring with NICHD, NIDA and NINDS. Using aMRI (anatomic Magnetic Resonance Imaging) DTI (Diffusion Tensor Imaging) and MRS (Magnetic Resonance Spectroscopy) to create a large scale data base of the normal brain development in children. The study is to reveal the development of circuitry for language, thinking and associated functions.

The Frontal Lobe of the brain is responsible for reasoning, planning, parts of speech, movement, emotion and problem solving. The Temporal Lobe of the brain is responsible for perception and recognition of sounds and memory.

University of North Carolina Medical School study concluded that by the age of two years children with Autism show an enlargement in the size of their brains. Scientists have not been able to explain the reason behind the approximately five percent greater brain growth but it has been suggested that the increased brain growth took place towards the child's first year of life.

STAART (Study To Advance Autism Research and Treatment) conducted MRI scans on Autistic and non Autistic two year old children. Having analysed brain tissue both grey and white they discovered significant enlargements across all regions in the Cerebral Cortex of Autistic children. Although the greatest volume increase was seen in the Temporal Lobe tissue enlargement was seen throughout the Cortex.

Summary

I am a mother of a fifteen year old Autistic boy. My child Steven was diagnosed as being severely Autistic with a severe receptive language disorder at two and a half years of age.

My book outlines the first hand experience that has been gained from my son Steven. The book has been written to assist and offer support to families, to create awareness of the subject of Autism and to demonstrate the complexities in brain development by comparing 'typical' development with 'Autistic' development.

The book covers the diagnostic process, concerns of parents, coping strategies, teaching methods, behaviour strategies, research being carried out on the subject, recognising educational needs, my child's developmental history and my approach to Autism. It also talks of finding an appropriate educational environment and offers practical guidance in this area. It offers guidance in teaching body awareness, developing life skills, building an understanding of the environment and everyday situations.

I gave up my career as an Interior Designer in Dubai to devote my time to Steven and used my creative skills to produce materials to further encourage his learning. I educated myself on the various strategies and the subject of Autism.

Seeing some progress in Steven's abilities, I returned to

the UK hoping it was the correct decision for him. Unfortunately, I have found that what I had hoped for Steven from the UK educational system wasn't what it turned out to be. I battled with the Local Education Authority to obtain the provision that Steven needed and felt frustrated at the lack of educational support that he received. Steven has been in an educational setting provided by the LEA for the past eight years and made no progress. Therefore, I have decided to teach him at home myself again on a full time basis. This is not an easy option for me but I feel that the system has failed him and I wish to provide Steven a chance to live and to show how much he is capable of achieving.

I will be picking up from where we left off when he was taught at home at the age of seven and through this book I want to help other parents to appreciate what they can achieve with their children through perseverance and love.

Sandy Howarth

GLOSSARY OF TERMS

Abnormal - Not normal. Deviating from the usual structure, condition and behaviour.

Absent spells - The individual experiencing the absent spell will appear to be staring into space.

Acetylcholine - A neurotransmitter which is responsible for transferring messages from one neuron to another.

Acquired - Which has been gained following an incident

ADHD (Attention Deficit and Hyperactivity Disorder) A condition that indicates a high level of activeness a lack of concentration and impulse control.

Amygdala - A part of the brain which plays a role in emotion

Annual review - A review of a special educational needs placement which must be carried out by the local education authority on 12 months of the statement being made or 12 months of the last review.

Anxiety - A mental health problem that causes the individual to experience a fear of a particular situation. People with Autism can express anxiety over things that most people see as every day living.

Anticonvulsant - a drug which is used to prevent and control seizures.

Antenatal - Conditions occurring before birth.

Auditory processing - The role in the brain which enables the function of hearing to develop learning. The ears play a part in sending messages while the hearing centers within the brain processes the information that has been received.

Auditory training - A form of Physical Therapy which uses a device to exercise the hearing apparatus, the ear drum, the ear bones and the cochlear membrane.

Aspraxia - A neurological speech disorder in which the child experiences difficulty in moving the muscles which are required for bringing out speech.

Articulation - The movement of the mouth, throat, tongue and teeth to form words

Audiologist - A medical professional who is trained to treat hearing loss and related disorders.

Auditory processing - The capacity of the brain to process information which has been heard which includes paying attention and responding to sounds, words or spoken language.

Autism - A neurological disorder, which affects an individual's development in areas of social, communication and imagination.

ASD - A term which is used when diagnosing a range of neurodevelopmental disorders which vary in the degree of severity. Autism is the severe form on the spectrum.

Asperger's Syndrome - An Autistic spectrum disorder which affects an individual's ability to relate to and communicate with others. Individuals with Asperger's Syndrome show average or above average intelligence and typical language development.

Assessment - A professional view of a child's needs to evaluate strengths, weaknesses and areas of difficulty. These include special educational needs, medical reports, a Speech Therapy report and a psychologist's report.

Bacteria - A single-celled micro organisms which exist

on its own or dependent on another organism for life

Biochemical - The application of chemistry to living things

Behavioural theory – The theory that Autism is a behavioral condition in which the behaviours stem from other underlying disorders which lead to the behaviours.

Beta endorphin - A hormone which is produced by the anterior pituitary gland which could affect memory. Beta endorphins can reduce the feeling of pain and affect feelings. When they are released in the body during exercise they are thought to cause the feeling of "runners high"

Brain - Part of the central nervous system. Its functions are to receive, process, organise and distribute information to the body. Consisting of two halves a left and right "hemispheres"

Brain stem - The lowest part of the brain which mergers with the spinal cord influencing basic processors such as alertness, breathing, blood pressure and heart rate.

Calcium - An essential mineral which is found in dairy products and green leafy vegetables. Calcium is a vital component in brain and muscle function as well as in overall health.

Carers - Members of the family, professionals and trained staff who provide constant care.

Casein - A protein which is found in cows milk and dairy products.

CAT scan - Images of structures within the body taken by a computer which turns multiple x-rays into visible images allowing 100% more clarity.

CDD (Childhood Disintegrative Disorder) - A disorder which indicates normal development in the first 24 months of life followed by rapid regression resulting in Autistic like symptoms.

Cerebellum - A part of the brain which sits above the brain stem and is responsible for coordination of movement and the function of balance. Known as the "little brain".

Cerebral - Referring to the brain, the cerebrum or intellect.

Cerebral cortex - The layer of the brain which is referred to as grey matter. It consists of bulges which add to the volume of its area whereby increasing the amount of information that can be processed. It is divided into right and left hemispheres, contains around two-thirds of the brain mass and covers most of the brain's structure.

Cerebral palsy - A chronic neurological disorder which affects the ability to control movements.

Chromosome 15 - One of the 23 pairs of chromosomes in human beings. A larger isodicentric chromosome 15 can cause poor muscle tone, mental retardation, behavioural problems and traits of Autism.

Code of practice - Offers guidance to LEAs schools and others involved in carrying out statutory duties.

Chromosome - A structure in the cell nucleus which is the carrier of genetic information. (46 chromosomes in a human being).

Cluster - A large number of decease which is concentrated in one area

Cognition - The ability to think, process, question and analyse.

Communication - The act of passing information from one to another.

Communication Disorder - Having difficulty using the typical methods of communication due to speech & language difficulties, loss of hearing or other neurological conditions.

Congenital Rubella Syndrome - A condition which usually manifests during infancy as a result of rubella infection. Symptoms include congenital glaucoma, congenital heart disease, loss of hearing, jaundice, microcephaly, mental retardation and bone disease.

Convulsions - Rapidly alternating contractions and relaxations of the muscles resulting the body to jerk uncontrollably.

Complex - Complicated and difficult to understand

Compromised - Unable to function efficiently with regard to the immune system.

Copper – An essential mineral which is necessary for overall health and enzyme function which is toxic when received in high doses.

Corpus Callosum - The major white matter tract of the brain which connects the left and right Cerebral hemispheres.

Craniosacral Manipulation - An alternative therapy in the treatment of Autism where the upper neck in moved by a qualified practitioner.

Cranium - Part of the skull which creates an enclosure to distinguish it from the face.

Deficiency - Having less than the required amount of one or more nutrients.

Degeneration - An alteration in the structure or chemical composition of tissue in which the function is interfered with by lowering its level of energy. Heredity plays a part in some cases.

Depression - A common mental health issue where the individual experiences   extreme sadness over a period of time.

Developmental Disorder - A disorder which interrupts the normal development process in childhood.

DFES - Department For Education and Skills.

DHA - An omega-3 essential fatty acid (EFA) which plays an important role in neurotransmission

Diagnose - The identification of a disorder which differentiates it from another to form an opinion of the nature of the illness.

DNA - Deoxyribonucleic acid - One of two types of molecules which contain genetic information. The other is RNA is transferred from it.

Dopamine - A chemical transmitter in the brain when released to the various areas in the brain acts as a pleasure producing substance. It is required in the normal functions of neurons and plays an important role of many functions within the nervous system which include mood, sleep, movement and motivation.

Dyslexia - A disorder which causes problems with learning to read.

Dyspraxia - A disorder which results in problems with planning and coordination.

Down Syndrome - A disorder which results in the child having 47 chromosomes instead of the expected 46 chromosomes. Associated with a distinct set of physical attributes together with a delay in learning abilities.

Early Intervention - The assessment and treatment of a child with a learning disability as early as possible, before the age of 4 years.

Echolalia - Repeating what has been said or heard in a parrot fashion.

EP (Educational Psychologist) - An individual involved in the assessment process of a child's special educational needs.

EEG - A test which places electrodes on the scalp to record electrical brain activity is used to detect seizures and abnormal brain activity. The brain experiences regular rhythmical changes of electrical potential due to the rhythmic discharge of energy by nerve cells. The changes are examined and recorded through graphic images.

EFA - Type of fatty acid which is essential in providing the required nutrients for the body and the brain.

EN2 Gene (Engrailed home-box 2) - Genes containing home box are said to play a part in controlling development.

Box Enzymes - Complex proteins which are produced by living cells present in digestive fluid in many tissues.

Endorphins - An opium like substance in the brain with painkilling and tranquilising properties.

Environmental triggers - Factors in the surrounding which could have an impact on development.

Etiology - The origin or cause of a disease. Scientists are studying the causes of Autism but no single identifiable cause has been found.

Expressive language - The ability to express ones thoughts verbally or non verbally.

Facial recognition - The ability to process and recognise through the faces of others of who they are.

Facilitated Communication - An approach which supports the child's wrist, arm or hand to assist communicate and spell words, phrases or sentences.

Fine motor skills - The ability to use the small muscles in the hands to manipulate and use   small items.

Floortime – A programme which focuses on encouraging meaningful interaction with children to enhance their emotional and social development. The name derives from the adults getting on the floor with children to participate in play activities.

Fragile X Syndrome – (FXS) The most common inherited form of mental retardation. Defined by gene changes in the FMR1 gene on the X chromosome. Approximately 25% of children with FXS have Autism.

Frontal Cortex – An area in the brain which is responsible for planning, movement, personality and intelligence. Judgment and impulse control also takes place in this region.

Frontal Lobe - The most anterior part of the cerebral cortex which is responsible for speech, movement, emotion, problem solving and personality.

Gastrointestinal - The stomach and small and large intestines.

Gene - The basic biological unit of heredity. 50,000-100,000 in human beings. They are located along the 23 pairs of chromosomes and similarly arrive in pairs. Humans possess 46 chromosomes. They consist of 2 sex chromosomes and 44 autosomes.

Generalisation - A form of developing skills not only through therapy but during activities performed in a variety of settings.

Genetic disorder - A disorder caused by abnormalities in the genes or chromosomes.

Gene splicing - The process of cutting the DNA of a gene using chemicals called restriction enzymes to act as scissors while adding the new DNA in its place.

Genetics - Recognised by genes and chromosomes.

Gluten free - A dietary intervention used in the treatment of Autism where all food containing gluten (barley, rye, oats and wheat) are removed from the diet.

Gross motor skills - The use of the large muscles in the body to perform actions and movements.

Grand mal seizure - A seizure which involves loss of consciousness with violent muscle contractions. The abnormal brain activity is experienced in the entire brain resulting in violent spasm throughout the body. Also known as tonic-clonic seizure.

Heredity - The various unusual features of bodily form, structure, physical features and mental activity transferred from the parents to the off spring.

High functioning - Refers to a higher level of skill in individuals with an impairment. For example, an Autistic person with good communication and appropriate behavior will be classed as a high functioning.

Hippocampus - A part of the brain involved in spatial orientation where information is processed. An area responsible for processing memories.

Hormones - Chemical messengers dispersed by the blood which act on organs to create effects which are different to the point of its release. They work slowly and over time affect different processors within the body. These include: growth and development, metabolism, sexual function, reproduction and mood. Hormones are powerful as it takes a small amount to cause major changes in the cells and the body. Therefore, too much or too little of a hormone can have serious effects.

HOXA1 Gene - A gene which plays a vital role in early mental development. The dysfunction of this gene is potentially related to traits detected in individuals with Autism.

IEP - Individual Education Plan - a written document which is prepared by professionals involved in the child's education together with the support of the parents which sets out targets to meet short term objectives.

Immune system - A system which distinguishes everything that is foreign and protects an individual against infections.

Immunisation - The introduction of antigen into the body to help provide immunity against various conditions.

Imagination - The ability to form a mental image of something which is not present by using ones mind.

Impairment - A lack of ability to function normally.

Inappropriate - Which is not suitable or acceptable.

Infection - the way in which a disease is transferred from one individual to another via micro organisms.

Intervention – A programme developed to help an individual with health and behavioural issues.

Integration - A process of educating special needs children where they are introduced to a full school curriculum mixing with normal role models.

Intonation - Speech consisting of changes in pitch and stress in the voice.

Language - Spoken, written or signed. Sounds and symbols grouped together to create meaningful words and words are grouped together to create meaningful sentences.

LEA - Local Education Authority - Part of the local

council which is responsible for providing education, assessing and maintaining statements.

Limbic system - The parts of the limbic system play an essential role in the normal expression of emotion, motivated behaviour and memory.

Lovaas Method - An intensive Behaviour Therapy programme created to teach Autistic children based on the theories of Professor Ivor Lovaas.

Magnesium – A mineral which is required for the health of every cell in the body.

Melatonin - A hormone which plays a part in the diurnal (night & day) function of the body. It derives from serotonin and is found in the pineal gland.

Memory - The capacity to process, register, store and recall which occurs in many regions of the brain including the limbic system.

Mental illness - A term used to describe a severe mental disorder which is recognised by a psychiatrist.

Metabolism - A range of biochemical processors which takes place within our system to break down food to transform into energy.

Met Gene - A gene which isn't specifically a brain gene where it affects multiple areas in the body including the function of the immune system. The connection between Autism and the MET gene has suggested that the condition may not be solely associated with brain development as previously believed.

Mind - Which thinks, feels reasons and perceives. In neuroscience the mind and body are one.

Migraine - Periodic attacks of headaches accompanied by nausea, vomiting and increased sensitivity of the eyes.

Mirror neurons - Neurons which are activated in the brain upon observation of another individual performing an action.

Motivational Techniques - Therapy that involves capitalising on the child's interests to motivate the child to respond.

Motor cortex - Areas of the Cerebral cortex which are responsible for the planning, control and execution of motor functions.

MMR vaccination - A combined vaccination which offers protection against measles, mumps and rubella (German measles)

MRI (Magnetic Resonance Imaging) - A technique which uses the magnetic qualities of chemicals in the body to produce an image of the brain

Neuroimaging - All forms of viewing neural activity through MRI scans PET scans or other.

Neurons - Cells that communicate throughout the body and the brain through electrical and biochemical signals.

Neurologist - A specialist in diagnosing and treating conditions associated with the nervous system.

Neuropsychological - A science which combined neurology and psychology to study the relationship between the central nervous system, the brain and behaviour.

Neurotransmitter - A substance such as dopamine or serotonin which is responsible for sending messages from one nerve cell to another by an electrical impulse.

Neurotypical - An individual who is neurologically normal.

Non verbal Communication - Communication which is recognised through the use of facial expression, body language, posture and the use of gestures.

Nutrition - The science and practice of taking in and utilising food.

OCD - Obsessive compulsive disorder. An anxiety disorder which is distinguished by recurring thoughts which are difficult to stop.

Onset - The first recognition of symptoms of an illness.

Omega-3 – Essential fatty acids which is found in fish and other foods seen as critical in brain function.

OT - Occupational therapist. A licensed therapist who provides help with developing life skills.

Paediatrician - A doctor who specialises in treating children.

Plastic – In biology, it refers to the changeability in living things such as the brain which can adjust and adapt. For example, an Autistic teenager who learns new skills suggests their brain is plastic.

PECS - Picture Exchange Communication System - A communication programme where the individual uses pictures to communicate a need.

Peptides - compound which is formed through the combination of two or more amino acids.

Petit Mal Seizure - Known as absence seizure, which is indicated through a sudden loss of consciousness. They are brief and can indicate staring spells, lip smacking and the fluttering of eye lids.

PET scan - A method used to measure mental activity in a particular area of the brain when performing a mental task.

Pragmatics - Study of language related to the structure and use.

Prevalence - The percentage of a population that has been diagnosed with a disease during a certain time.

Proposed statement - A statement of educational needs issued by the LEA in draft form before it has been agreed and finalised.

Psychiatry - The branch of medical science which is involved in the treatment and management of mental illness and help in the area of learning disabilities.

Purkinje cells - A lack of Purkinje cells in the brain has been associated with Autism.

Receptive language - The ability to interpret language received verbally and non verbally.

Receptors – Proteins that are attached to the surface of the cell which receive biochemical messages from the body. Cell receptors are essential in communication between brain cells and other cells in the body.

Regression - Loss of previously acquired skills.

Respite - Short term care provided for individuals with disabilities to offer a break to the care givers.

Retts Syndrome - A neurological disorder which affects only girls.

Ritalin - (Methylphenidate) is a stimulant used in treating ADHD (Attention Deficit & Hyperactivity Disorder)

Savant abilities - An Autistic individual who shows extreme talent in one specific area.

Scan - An image obtained by examining the areas of the body by using a sensing device.

Secretin - A hormone which has been used to detect signs of problems related to the digestive system.

Self injurious Behaviour - A self directed behaviour which causes physical damage to the individual exhibiting the behaviour.

SENCO - Special Education Needs Coordinator - A member of staff of a school who is responsible for coordinating the special educational needs.

Sensory integration - A neurological ability to gather and process accurately information received through our senses.

Serotonin – A chemical which is a neurotransmitter in the central nervous system. Recognised as the "feel good chemical" which has a profound effect on mood and anxiety.

Shared attention - Both play partners focus their attention on the same thing.

Side effects - Problems resulting from a treatment which goes beyond the desired effect.

Sign Language - A method of communication using hands to support language use and understanding of speech.

Sleep - The body's rest cycle

Social behavior - The ability to establish and maintain satisfactory interpersonal skills displaying behaviour within social expectations while possessing the ability to make personal adjustments.

Somatosensory Cortex - The area in the brain which detects tactile stimulation which include touch, temperature, pain, itch and tickles together with muscle movement, joint position, facial expression and sensory information within the body.

Speech Therapy - Delivered by a trained professional who will assist in diagnosing and treating developmental and communication disorders.

Statementing - The preparation of a formal document which specifies additional support required to meet a child's special educational needs.

Statutory assessment - A formal procedure carried out by the Local Education Authority, which involves a detailed assessment of the child's special educational needs, and the provision required to meet those needs.

Stereotypical Behaviour - Behavior which is repeated many times over.

Stim - Self stimulation as a way of stimulating ones senses.

Sub Clinical Seizure - A seizure which indicates a trace of abnormal brain activity when observed through an EEG. Though, it doesn't correspond with the level of consciousness in the individual. It lasts for a short period of time and does not show any obvious signs of clinical symptoms.

Temporal Lobe - An area in the brain which is a part of the Cerebrum. It plays a vital role in language and vision. In addition it contains the hippocampus where it is involved with memory formation.

Theory of mind deficit - The theory that people with Autism lack the basic understanding of beliefs, thoughts, knowledge and ideas of others.

Triad of impairments - Autism is recognised by the triad of impairments which affects areas of social, communication and imagination.

Tribunal hearing - A meeting where an appeal is considered.

Tuberous Sclerosis - A rare genetic disorder which results in the growth of benign tumours within the brain and or other organs such as kidneys, lungs, heart, eyes and the skin.

Tactile - Related to touch

TEACCH - Treatment and Education of Autism and related Communication Children Handicapped - A whole life approach to teaching children and adults with Autistic spectrum disorders.

Therapy -The treatment of an illness

Theory of mind - The ability to recognise that another person has an individual perspective which is different to ones own.

Time out -A procedure where the child is removed from a setting for a specific period of time without any positive reinforcement.

Visual Schedule - A schedule which consists of photographs, pictures, written words or objects. It's prepared for an individual with a communication disorder to help understand a series of activities.

AUTISM REFERENCE - 1
RECOMMENDED READING – BOOKS

- The Autistic Spectrum - (A guide for parents and professionals) Lorna Wing
- The world of the Autistic child - Bryna Siegel
- Behaviour Intervention for young children with Autism (Catherine Maurice, Gina Green & Steven C.Luce
- Autism - Professional perspectives and practice - Chapman & Hall
- Understanding and Teaching children with Autism - Rita Jordan & Stuart Powell
- Children with Autism - A parents' guide
- Somebody somewhere - Donna Williams
- Autism and Learning (A guide to good practice) Stewart Powell and Rita Jordan

1. AUTISM - CAUSES

- Autism
- Autism causes and what you can do to help reverse it (Healthreports.com)

2. AUTISM & RELATED DISORDERS

- Centre for study of Autism
- Autism, Asperger's Syndrome and Semantic pragmatic disorder: Where are the boundaries
- Childhood epilepsy - Autism

3. RESEARCH

- Autism reveals social roots of language
- Brain function of individuals diagnosed with Autism during emotion discrimination
- An exciting new theory regarding the cause of Autism (Autism@rollingdigital.com)
- Autism FAQ - Well known research and practitioners

- The cerebellum and Autism (Centre for the study of Autism)
- Autism Research Centre
- The analysis of Autism facilitates neuroanatomical investigations
- BBC New / Health - Differences found in the Autistic brain
- Autistic brain not damaged where researchers expected (scienceandtechnology@scientificamerican.com)
- Research - Autistic children's brains grow larger during first years of development
  (UNC News release)
- New releases - Deciphering a mystery (Society of Neuroscience)
- Research finds size differences in the brains of autistic individuals
- What's going on in the Autistic brain?
- Autistic spectrum disorders (Research at the National Institute of Mental Health)
- Autism Research Centre - What is Autism?
- How does the Autistic brain work (Closer to the truth)
- New device will help people with Autism relate to those around them (Autism Connect)
- Autism speaks launches campaign to research causes (Autism Connect)
- Weak brain links may explain Autism (Autism Connect)
- People with Autism are more intelligent than previously thought (Autism Connect)
- Potential of people with Autism is unlimited (Autism Connect)

4. AUDITORY & SENSORY INTEGRATION

- The American Occupational Therapy association (AOTA consumers tip sheets)
- Sensory integration dysfunction - Interview with Carol Kranowitz (Author of out of sync child)
  Sensory integration international - Frequently asked questions FAQ Centre
- Sensory integration diagnosis, causes, symptoms and treatments
- Auditory integration training

5. LIVING, LOVING & LEARNING

6. SOCIAL BEHAVIOUR IN AUTISM / SOCIAL SKILLS TRAINING

- Social skills in children with Autism: Development and training
- Social behaviour in Autism (Centre for the study of Autism)
- Understanding behaviour through social & emotional development (Centre for the study of Autism)
- Autism & emotions (neurodiversity.com)
- Anxiety, fears & phobias
- Emotional competence in children with Autism spectrum disorder
- Social problems: Understanding emotions & developing talents (Centre for the study of Autism)

7. CONTROVERSIES

- Autism FAQ - Controversies
- Controversies in Autism - Wikipedia

8. THINKING & DEVELOPING CONCENTRATION

- Thinking of thinking as a hobby - (Autism Diva)

9. IMMUNISATIONS / DRUGS / HEALTH

- Vitamin B6 and magnesium (Centre for the study of Autism)
- BBC Health - Conditions - Autism
- Autism spectrum disorders (Health)
- Misconceptions about immunisation
- Hearing information on Health line
- Views from the Autistic spectrum and the psychiatrist
- AMJ psychiatry
- Autism and vaccination
- British government accused of inexplicable complacency

over MMR vaccine (Autism Connect)
- Panel discussion of vaccine safety opens upcoming Autism conference
- Action for Autism - MMR Rant

AUTISM REFERENCE -2

1. STRUCTURED TEACHING

- Structured Teaching - Autism
- Start-up program

2. UNDERSTANDING THE THEORY OF MIND

- Experience with visual thinking, sensory problems and communications difficulties Temple Grandin (Centre for the study of Autism)
- Theory of mind - Wikipedia
- The Autistic mind
- Understanding Autism - The physiological basis and biomedical intervention options of Autism spectrum disorders
- Does the Autistic child have a theory of mind?
- Theory of mind
- Mind information - booklets by series
- Left brain / right brain

3. TREATMENTS & APPROACHES

- Public Autism awareness (Autism Interventions)
- Autism FAQ treatment
- Treatment - Cure Autism now
- Strategies for teaching children with Autistic spectrum disorders
- Autism software - teaching tips
- Teaching good communication skills

- Treatment strategies for children with social cognitive deficits including Aspergers,
- Autism, PDD, NLD, ADHD
- Teaching tips for children and adults with Autism
- Temple Grandin (Centre for the study of Autism)
- Rethinking Autism /PDD
- Autism software - Teaching tips
- Parent tips for working with teachers

4. TEMPLE GRANDIN - THINKING IN PICTURES

- Autism current issues - Mike Connor
- The culture of Autism
- Thinking in pictures - Autism and visual thought - Expanded edition

5. STRESS & COPING / FAMILIES

- Parents of children with Autism
- Physician to parent - sharing concerns
- Current strategies for coping with an Autistic child in the family (Mike Connor)
- Advice for the parent who just discovered their child is Autistic
- Autistic need best support
- Coping (Autism FAQ)
- About Autism - Why me?
- Aunty Blabby - A helpful exercise for siblings (Centre for the study of Autism)
- Factors associated with functioning style and coping strategies of families with ASD
- Tips for a person with Aspergers Syndrome
- Stress on families (www.patient enters.com)
- Sibling issues
- Stress on families (Autism Society of America)
- The Autistic family life cycle: Family - Stress and divorce
- ASA's 37th National conference on Autism

6. BOOKS / DVDS / VIDEOS

- Book reviews - Could it be Autism
- Monarch educational - materials
- Preparing for first grade
- Developing gross motor skills
- Modelling good hygiene habits
- Skills your child will learn watching physical power - Activity videos
- Promoting self - reliance
- Exercising fine motor muscles
- Practicing dressing skills
- Strengthening concentration
- Improving hand eye coordination
- Boosting self confidence
- MT & Autism

AUTISM REFERENCE - 3

1. AUTISM GENERAL

- Autism crisis; The facts (The Observer / politics)
- Autism & PDD (Squirrel mail)
- Pervasive developmental disorders : Autism
- Aspergers Syndrome and ASD (National Autistic Society)
- Autism in children
- The Autistic mind by Gary Waleski
- What causes Autism
- Autism fact sheet
- Children & Adolescents with Autism (National Mental Health Information Centre)
- Parent's questions (Centre for the study of Autism)
- Autism - Yale development disabilities clinic
- Autism - Nemours foundation

2. THERAPIES

- Communication in Autism
- Speech & Language therapy, speech information on Autism and disorders
- Autism treatment trust
- Frequently asked questions
- A program for children challenged by Autism - for parents and children
- Autistic children make progress with play (squirrel mail)
- Autism treatments, interventions & findings
- Teaching Autistic children who aut to be home
- The use of diet and vitamins in the treatment of Autism (The NAS)
- Autism FAQ - Educational methods
- Autism Web - Educating children with Autism & PDD
- Autism therapies & approaches
- Therapies (Aspies for freedom)
- Behaviour modification - The Lovaas method autism Research Institute

3. BEHAVIOUR / DIAGNOSIS

- So your child was just diagnosed
- Diagnosis (Autism for parents)
- Chapter 111 - Early identification of young children with possible Autism
- Autism: Recognising the signs in young children
- Toe walking (Centre for the study of Autism)
- Autism medication: Treating self stimulation, and other Autistic behaviour
- Characteristic behaviour (Autism FAQ)
- Autism - Repetitive behaviour & obsessions - The story of Temple Grandin

4. BIOMEDICAL APPROACHES

- Some biomedical approaches to Autism

5. DRUGS

- Pharmacotherapy & Autism: References

6. EMOTIONS

- Social problems: understanding emotions and developing talents (Temple Grandin)
- Learning to smile
- The theoretical use of the affective trigger as a tool for the emotional education of Children with developmental impairments
- Science daily: In Autism & related disorders recognising emotion is different than identity
- Understanding behaviour through social - emotional development (Centre for the Study of Autism)
- Autism & Emotions - (www.neurodiversity.com/autism&emotions)

7. SURVIVAL GUIDE FOR PEOPLE ON THE AUTISTIC SPECTRUM

8. LIVING WITH AUTISM / DIAGNOSIS

- Screening for Autism
- Autism guide - Stress on families with Autistic children
- Autism for parents
- Autism guide - living with Autism - overview
- Autism information library - What is Autism like for those who have it?
- Physical examination for Autism

9. FAMILY / CAREGIVING

- Adolescents and adults with Autism - A study of family care giving

AUTISM REFERENCE - 4

1. ACTION FOR AUTISM / CONTROVERSIES

- To argue or not to argue - (Centre for the study of Autism)
- The infamous cure debate
- Autism - Lord Hansard (United Kingdom parliament)
- Action for Autism - MMR rant
- Autism bulletin
- Controversies in Autism - (Wikipedia)
- Controversies about functioning labels in the Autistic spectrum (Wikipedia)
- New study: MMR link to the onset of Autism? The debate continues (Blogcadre)
- Panel discussion of vaccine safety opens upcoming Autism conference
- Drinking coffee will not make your child Autistic (Autism vox)
- Action for Autism - Where is the debate
- Sunday times (Squirrel mail)
- Tree house policy and campaigns
- Action for Autism - Mike Stanton (Squirrel mail)

2. EDUCATIONAL ISSUES / DIAGNOSIS

- Genius may be an abnormality (Centre for the study of Autism)
- Educational methods - (Autism FAQ)
- After the IEP is in place - Educational issues (www.parentcenters.com)
- Tip sheets Autism - (AOTA)
- Find a therapist (Health)

3. SEN / CODE OF PRACTICE

- Autism FAQ - Advocacy
- UK Educational statementing process
- Shaping the future of Special Education - An action program for Wales
- SEN code of practice on the identification and assessment of pupils with special Educational needs

4. CASE STUDIES

- Using creative expertise to help pupils with Autistic spectrum disorder
- Neuro feedback treatment - Review of 60 cases
- A case study on Autism: School accommodations and inclusive settings
- Best practice - case study - A young child who has literacy and also has Autism
- Special connections - Case study summaries

5. THEORY OF AUTISM

- What they aren't telling you about Autism - Comments on this unique theory

6. GENE MAY CAUSE AUTISM

- Gene may cause Autism - study (Medi 4 - dispatch online)
- Autism is likely to be linked to several genes (American psychological association)
- Sever Autism spectrum disorder could be reversible
- Gene breakthrough holds key to cure Autism (Cure Autism now AGRE)
- A promising Autism breakthrough (Newsweek Health - MSNBC.com)
- BBC News - Autism gene breakthrough hailed
- Gene therapy breakthrough for Autism condition

- Researchers discover first Autism susceptibility gene

7. RESEARCH

- The international Autism Research Organisation
- Autism Victoria - Research - Get involved
- How does the Autistic brain work? (Closer to the truth - show 3)
- Advice for parents of young children with Autism (Autism Research Institute)
- Scientific foundations of a DAN protocol (Autism Research Institute)
- Positive outcome with neurofeedback treatment in case of mild Autism
- Autism - New study - MMR link to onset of Autism (Blogcadre)
- Autism Research at the NICHD

8. NEWS

9. NEWS / FAMOUS AUTISTIC PEOPLE / NAS / INCLUSIVE TECHNOLOGY

- People speculated to have been Autistic
- The National Autistic Society - What the NAS does
- Inclusive technology

<u>INDEX</u>
(All main headings have been written in bold)

NO MATTER WHAT

Lightning Source UK Ltd.
Milton Keynes UK
19 January 2011
165970UK00001B/5/P